The Goddess D.I.E.T.

SEE A GODDESS IN THE MIRROR IN 21 DAYS

Published by	Now Age Publishing Pty Ltd PO Box 1800, Margaret River, Western Australia 6285 NowAgePublishing.com
Cover by	Inspired Insight inspired-insight.com
Cover image	Stefan Muran
Back cover image	Marie-Lan Nguyen / Wikimedia Commons
Printed in Australia	

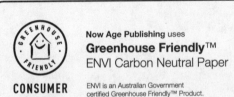

GREENHOUSE FRIENDLY

CONSUMER

Now Age Publishing uses
Greenhouse Friendly™
ENVI Carbon Neutral Paper

ENVI is an Australian Government
certified Greenhouse Friendly™ Product.

The text for this book has been printed on carbon neutral paper

National Library of Australia Cataloguing-in-Publication entry

Author:	Revel, Anita, 1968-
Title:	The goddess diet : see a goddess in the mirror in 21 days / Anita Revel.
Edition:	1st ed.
ISBN:	9780980443912 (pbk.)
Notes:	Includes index. Bibliography.
Subjects:	Mind and body. Body image. Self-care, Health. Spiritual life.
Dewey Number:	158

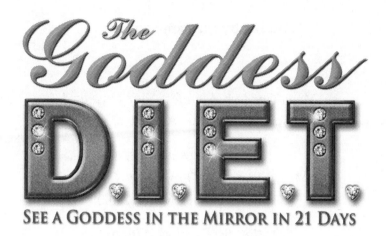

The Goddess D.I.E.T.

SEE A GODDESS IN THE MIRROR IN 21 DAYS

ANITA REVEL

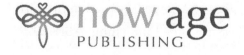
now age
PUBLISHING

Books by the same author

Moon Goddess, Manifest Your Dreams
(Goddess.com.au   August 2006)

Selena's Crystal Balls,
A Magical Journey Through the Chakras
(Goddess.com.au   March 2007)

Outing the Goddess Within,
One Girl's Journey With 52 Guides
(Goddess.com.au   January 2008)

The 7-Day Chakra Workout
(ChakraGoddess.com April 2008)

Sacred Vigilance, Wide-Awake Meditation
(Goddess.com.au   September 2008)

Goddess At Play, A Journal For Self-Discovery and Play
(Goddess.com.au   February 2009)

What Would Goddess Do?
A Journal for Channelling Divine Guidance
(Goddess.com.au   March 2009)

The Goddess Guide to Chakra Vitality, 3rd Edition
(Now Age Publishing April 2009)

Praise for The Goddess DIET

What a fabulous, illuminated and wise guide The Goddess DIET is! This is exactly the kind of support and inspiration we want and need.

SARK, PlanetSARK.com

Brimming with fun, wit and compassion, Anita Revel will inspire you to step into the beautiful body that is your birthright. She is the cheerleader you've been waiting for!

Regena Thomashauer (aka Mama Gena), founder of Mama Gena's School of Womanly Arts.

Written with her usual blend of wit and wisdom, Anita Revel cuts to the core to get your inner goddess fit, feisty and fabulous. This book is stuffed with sound advice, illuminating stories and womanly wisdom.

Dr Sharon Turnbull, author of Goddess Gift: Discover Your Personal Goddess Type.

The Goddess DIET is an intriguing roadmap to reveal the sassy, powerful and divine goddess in us all. It serves up a delightful combination of insight, inspiration and ideas to reveal your best you. A must for those seeking a dose of all three.

Kristen Schuerlein, founder of Affirmagy.

I encourage you to let Anita guide you on your quest to re-shape your precious mind, body and spirit in positive and beautiful new ways.

Lucy Cavendish, author of Wild Wisdom of the Faery.

Anita has shown me how to heal my own ego with a concept so simple it was right before my eyes.

Charmaine Wilson, winner of The One and author of Spirit Whispers.

Understanding the body/mind/spirit connection is essential on the path of self-love. Recommended reading for all present and future self-proclaimed goddesses.

J. Alison Hilber, author of Change the Way You See.

The Goddess DIET is not a stereotypical program. Instead it is a body-mind-spirit plan to uncover the goddess within. Reveal a new, healthier, more confident and vibrant you, and the passion to let your true self shine.

Serene Conneeley, author of Seven Sacred Sites: Magical Journeys That Will Change Your Life.

It's no doubt that The Goddess DIET is an amplified offering of Anita Revel's "go get 'em" energy.

Maria Elita, author of The Miracle.

I've been every size from 6 to 18, and have slowly come to accept my body as the manifestation of the Goddess in all her forms. Anita Revel's 21-day plan is an inspiring and fun way to get there.

Joanne Lock, Co-founder of Spellcraft Magazine, Australia

This book will delight you. The hard facts are well researched, the inspiration is spot-on and the humour, as always, helps the medicine go down.

Elizabeth Stephens, author of Seven Angels Helped Me – They'll Help You Too

I love Anita's clever turning of the usual self-loathing diet program into the self-loving 'Goddess in the Mirror' we can all become.

Carolinda Witt, author of T5T: The Five Tibetan Exercise Rites

The Goddess DIET inspires and empowers you to realign your outer self with your inner self. You'll love the side-effects!

Nicole Graham, co-creator of Journal for the Modern Goddess.

This project has been created with love,
for wise women every where,
every age, every body,
every stage.

Love love love,
Anita Revel
April 2009

Warning: Possible Side-Effects

Before undertaking The Goddess DIET, be warned that the following side-effects have been reported by women who have completed the program:

✻ Inexplicable desires to dance;

✻ Bursts of random happiness;

✻ Outbreaks of outrageous luck;

✻ Unsolicited acts of kindness to self;

✻ Eruptions of revived passion for living;

✻ Frequent glimpses of your inner wow factor;

✻ Spontaneous bouts of smiling for no reason;

✻ Unprecedented feelings of self-respect;

✻ Unintentional moments of cheerfulness;

✻ Easy-peasy weight regulation;

✻ Effortless energy throughout the day;

✻ Irresistible attraction to love and light;

✻ Multitudes of women asking for your secret;

✻ Earth-shattering sense of peace and well-being;

✻ Holistic health in all aspects of your life.

Disclaimer: Please do not purchase or share this book unless you are prepared to accept and relish the consequences as outlined above.

Dear Goddess... a Note From the Author

If you're reading this book because you think it's a manual for weight-loss, it's my guess you:

  a) *think* you're fat;
  b) really are fat;
  c) both of the above.

Take heart. If you are conditioned to be ashamed of your curves (as I was when I started this program), well, it's time to overhaul your thinking about dieting, your body, your body image, your self esteem and your holistic well-being. It's time to get *real*.

It is my pleasure to redefine the concept of dieting by providing you with **D**aily **I**ntentional **E**mpowerment **T**ools ('DIET') to help you feel good about yourself. No more dangerous dieting; no more trash talking; no more self-loathing... The Goddess DIET realigns your physical, emotional and spiritual behaviours so that you can see a goddess in the mirror within 21 days.

When I first developed The Goddess DIET in 2005, my initial goal was to get back into my bikini. Happily, this program taught me so much more about myself and my values so that eventually, the bikini became a non-issue – I soon realised it was my *attitude* that was keeping me in the loop of self-loathing.

So, this project is the result of my decision to change my life in order to regain it. Physically, I found the ideal weight for my body (and my wardrobe!) that is sustainable, healthy and keeps me energised. And although I did lose a dress size as a side-effect of respecting my body, I attained so much more than a simple diet plan could have given me – I also benefited enormously on emotional and spiritual levels too. I lost my inner critic, gained more energy and fell in self-love.

Nearly four years on, I'm still living The Goddess DIET with ease. In fact, even though I'm a rampant foodie, regard champagne as a major food group, and have a new baby at the time of completing this book, I'm still lighter, healthier and happier than ever before.

I recorded the journey so you can see that even someone with a history of bulimia and chronic lethargy can overcome ingrained self-loathing and see a goddess in the mirror in 21 days. Herewith, is my journey, 'warts', tantrums, tiaras and all.

Love and light refreshments,

Anita
xx

Anita Revel

Menu of Delectable Insights

Part 1: Getting Ready

Part 1:

Getting Ready

The 'Before' Shot

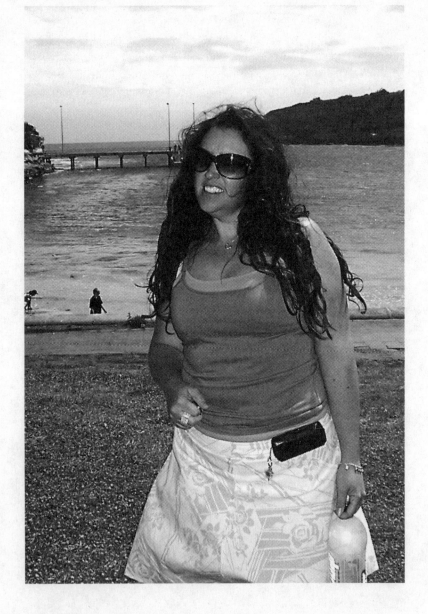

Bloated and zapped… Anita looking for a nap at Childer's Cove while asking herself, "Where did these D-Cups come from?"

In The Beginning...

This journey all started when I looked in the mirror to discover I had the body of a god. Yeah, Buddha. With my 159cm frame carrying 70 kilograms I felt zapped, lazy and totally peeved off that my wardrobe no longer fit me. Perhaps worst of all, I had lost my libido at around the extra-six-kilograms mark. It went out the window along with my aspirations to get another season out of my bikini. By the time I'd piled on 12 kilograms in as many months, my energy levels had plummeted, my eyes had resilient black bags, my hair was on a permanent bad day, and I felt like I was living in a foggy tunnel. The day I passed out from sheer exhaustion was a neon sign that it was time to reverse the trend. Although I hadn't spilled a drop of my Cosmopolitan at the time, I wasn't proud of who I was or how I was no longer in control of my body.

It wasn't just my comfort level that had me reaching for the diet books. It was my energy levels I was most worried about, along with my declining zest for life. I had lost my spark, my zing, my love for dancing to 80s music. I needed a plan that would get me back to where I used to be – a walking disco ball of sparkle and *joie de vivre*.

Sadly, I found all the diets I researched were one-dimensional in their approach to weight-loss. They were about discipline, sacrifice and treadmills – all dirty words in my vocabulary. That's when I came up with The Goddess DIET – a complete program that addresses not just the physical body, but also the mind and the spirit.

Many traditional diets promise you will lose a few kilos in a few weeks. Dangerous diets promise more than that. All diets are usually fussy or extreme, and you're expected to fit the preparation of special foods into your busy lifestyle.

The Goddess DIET is a little different. Your 'weight' loss happens when you chuck out the extra baggage you've been carrying needlessly. And you will get to know your 'thinner goddess' when you purify your attitude to your self-image, your approach to life, and the decisions you make every day to honour your goddess within.

This 'diet' (for want of a better four-letter word) is an holistic approach to well-being using a variety of tools that are already at your fingertips. It's just a matter of using them. Perhaps what makes my plan so special is that it can be incorporated into your daily life – so much so, even the husband and kids can join in too (and they don't even have to know!).

I wish to emphasise that the intention of The Goddess DIET is not to make you a size zero, celebrity rich or peachy popular. The goal of this DIET is to be able to look into a mirror and be wowed by the woman you see in the glass.

This means being comfortable in your skin (regardless of the size on the tag of your jeans), empowered in your choices, and feeling at ease with who you are as a goddess.

The 'Forever-After' Shot

Nearly four years on, Anita is still lighter (of mind and body), happier and more energetic than ever before.

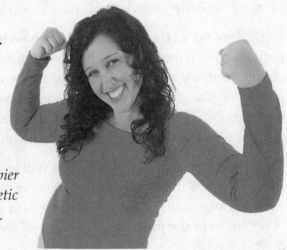

Good Riddance to Bad Habits

Before you start your own Goddess DIET, it's a good idea to review your current lifestyle and prepare for the new. Throw out your old addictions, bad habits and obsessive and automatic behaviours. This does not need to be difficult, as I shall explain.

Think about your life right now. You wake up, groan as you open the curtains, waddle on auto-pilot to the kettle, make coffee, drink coffee, think about how you need more coffee… and all this before you get the kids up, get them ready for school, get yourself ready for work, think about the list of jobs to do as you drive the same route every day, absent-mindedly wave the kids off to their classrooms… the list goes on. Pretty predictable, right?

Well, no more Ms Predictable. The Goddess DIET requires that you step outside of your daily mondo for 21 days so that you can bury old habits. Or at least retire them. So go to your diary right now and circle the day you will be staring your transformation. Step aside Ms Boring-Routine, and welcome Ms Fabulous-Divine-Look-At-Me-Super-Booty-Luscious-Wonder-Goddess.

Why 21 Days?

Thanks to the work by plastic surgeon Dr Maxwell Maltz in the 1950s and '60s, it is now accepted that it takes 21 days to break a habit. This came about when Dr Maltz noticed his patients would often feel the same on the inside even if they'd had reconstructive surgery to look different on the outside. He realised that a person's relationship with their inner-self self paves the way for how they see their outer-self, so in an effort to avoid the scalpel, set about improving self-image as a means to repairing the patient's outer-self.

Upon further investigation, he noted in his book, *Psycho-Cybernatics* (Pocket Books 1971), that it took 21 days for amputees to cease 'feeling' their amputated limb. He applied the same 21-day window to create self-image improvement prior to surgery, with the result being surgery became unnecessary for many patients.

Dr Maltz's 21-day theory was supported when Yale School of Medicine researchers looked closely at synaptic connections (the brain circuitry that allows brain cells to talk to each other). According to Charles Greer, professor of neurosurgery and neurobiology and senior author of the study[1], synaptic connections "...do not appear until 21 days after the birth of new brain cells."

While the new cells are maturing, they rely on signals from other brain regions thereby taking on existing patterns of behaviour. So by escaping your routine and applying new stimuli and data to your brain for 21 days straight, you are effectively training your new brain cells to behave in accordance with your new rules.

Science and research aside, I can vouch for the 21 day theory because it worked for me... which is why I'm recommending that you also commit 21 days to escaping routine. I went on a holiday to Tasmania to do it, but if you don't have any vacation time owing, don't worry. Just aim to mix up the daily grind a bit in order to get a new perspective on what's important.

It's not rocket science that if you make the same choices you get the same results. In fact, one of my favourite expressions during a brainstorming session is, "If you always do what you've always done, you'll always get what you've always got." So the key to breaking into new habits is to create new rules for yourself. Take a walk at the same time every day. Incorporate an apple into breakfast every day. Prepare for a meditation using the same ritual – wear the same clothes, burn the same oils, use the same relaxation technique before you begin. The more senses you can get involved the better. By your fourth week, you'll know you have been successful when it is easier to do the new behaviour than not to.

Alright, next step... now listen to what your sub-conscious is saying as you read that last paragraph. Is it along the lines of, "but I can't because..."? Goddess sister, I've heard all the excuses:

- I have to get little Johnny to school every day;
- Hubby expects me to do the daily household chores;
- My work deadlines are set in cement;
- My calendar is chock-a-block with commitments...

Fair enough, you're busy and have responsibilities. For some of us cramming every moment with an activity is what we thrive on. It helps keep our minds off the really important stuff, like... pampering ourselves, giving time to our true passions, resolving past hurts, revelling in our brilliance... Ah, but it all comes down to choice, doesn't it? For example;

- I can choose to spend six weekends organising little Johnny's fundraiser, or I can delegate and spend the salvaged time and energy on my own well-being;
- I can spend hours vacuuming, cleaning windows and making everyone's lunches, or I can teach my partner and kids to contribute to the household harmony;
- I can say "yes" to the boss every time additional expectations are dumped onto my desk, or I can teach one of my team members to do more in their role – it's a win-win situation in that they feel more empowered with their increased responsibility and role diversity, and I get to shine on with my job.

Or, I can continue believing that I simply need to keep pushing against the obstacles presenting themselves to me, and in doing so, continue achieving the same results of zero Me Time on one side of the scale, and ongoing exhaustion, resentment and isolation on the other.

All you need to do is change your response, behaviour or perspective to your perceived blockage in order to move onwards and upwards.

Sounds simple enough, but am I hearing you slip into the old habit of saying "it's toooo haaaaard"?

Some things are easy to change: you just do it. Other things are harder to change. Or are they just hard because you're conditioned to *believe* that they're hard? Why does it have to be hard? Why can't it be easy?

---

*If you catch yourself saying, "It's hard," stop and consciously change your statement to, "**It is easy**."*

It is easy

Feel how wonderfully easy everything appears after you've said it is easy! How easy is that?! Too easy ☺

It is not enough to *wish* you had 21 days to do this plan. It's not enough to sigh and say, "Well, I had good intentions to do The Goddess DIET, but it's not going to work out for me because…" (Here's where you wheel out the same tired old excuses that you've always used to limit your potential.) You must consciously choose to change your habitual responses to your blockages. That is, you can only change your blockages by changing your mind about how you will manage them.

Tips on Making Changes

You may feeling stuck in a rut, whether it be at work, home, or on the bathroom scales, but I want you to feel as young and energetic as the changes you make allow you to be. Success comes from being conscious of your choices, your reasons for making those choices, the insights that come from this consciousness, and how you apply new habits.

The first step in making change is self-examination – finding your triggers. Look at the way you react to situations in order to begin to understand your programming. When these situations arise again, and you can sense yourself stepping into a familiar behavioural pattern, you can then consciously choose to react or respond differently.

For example, before The Goddess DIET I had a pattern whereby at 8.30pm I would gravitate to the TV for whatever crime show was scheduled for that evening. I'd traipse upstairs with whatever was left in the wine bottle from dinner and sit in front of the TV with my husband until the bottle was finished (and beyond). When I self-examined this behaviour I realised I wasn't really interested in what was on TV, but this was a habit I'd developed to wind down, (which I affectionately refer to as wine-downing). I recognised this was unhealthy, not just because of the excessive amount of wine, but also because our relationship was sinking into the doldrums.

I consciously chose to change this pattern while I was on vacation in Tasmania and weaned myself off the nightly TV ritual. It was easy to do while on vacation when there were so many new things to see and do instead. When I returned home to Western Australia, I stocked the fridge with sparkling mineral water and at 8.30 each evening, I would drink that (in a champagne glass as part of my new ritual) instead of wine. Furthermore, hubby and I began to play backgammon instead of mindlessly tuning in to the TV. The upshot is that I gained clarity, slept better than ever, and our relationship got even stronger.

I am proud of my choice to change. I don't see it as *giving up* the TV ritual, but rather, I see it as *gaining* a new (and improved) ritual of sparkling mineral water in a flute glass, laughter and chit-chat over a mind-stimulating activity, and an enriched relationship with my man.

1. See Change as Positive

It's a trap to think that in order to change it requires sacrifice. Breaking bad habits is simply a positive step in taking care of yourself. From here on, you are adopting new habits that will serve you well for many years to come. You are honouring the beautiful being you were born to be. And you're leaving behind some unnecessary baggage and gaining fabulosity.

Hasta la vista	Hola!
Uggghhh in the mirror	Wolf whistles
Blotchy skin	10 years younger
Lank hair	Lustrous locks
Brittle fingernails	Strong, natural nails
Poor posture	Fashion model
Inadequacy	Control of your destiny
Feelings of self-loathing	Million dollar self-worth
Envy of social butterflies who are the centre of attention at parties and gatherings	The shining light that draws the butterflies (and the occasional beautiful moth) ;-)

2. Positive Reinforcement

While I'm a fan of positive reinforcement (rewarding good behaviour), some researchers say that penalties work just as well for changing behavioural patterns. You don't need to go so far as giving yourself an electric shock each time you transgress, but if you really are stuck in the self-flagellation mindset, try 'punishments' (ha ha) such as 10 sit-ups each ad-break, or 10 lunges between each glass of wine.

Be careful though, that you don't make misery a part of your routine. Happiness begets happiness. Misery only keeps you on the same old treadmill that got you miserable in the first place.

I believe that old-school religion has got a lot to do with the mindset that states, "If I suffer now I'll be rewarded with heavenly bliss later on." I've *never* understood this message – why can't we be happy now *and* happy later? Apply this thinking to The DIET, and ask yourself, "Why punish myself now for a future reward? Why not just find something I enjoy doing and do it always?" If pay-now-play-later is how you've been trained, again, I ask you to overhaul your thinking, your conditioning and the core values you have been taught, and consider *what is right for you.*

What is going to make your inner muse sing? What will you be able to maintain day-in and day-out because you *want* to, rather than because you *have* to. In other words, make choices for yourself that mean this DIET is enjoyable for you for a very long time.

Pssst. Reward good behaviour with 10 sit-ups each ad-break, or 10 lunges between the vegie chopping… You see where I'm heading with this? Punishment. Reward. Whatever… Just see exercise as fun!

3. Forgiveness

Janice Taylor, aka Our Lady of Weight Loss[2], has a slogan that I love: "All is forgiven. Move on."

"Forgiveness is a key ingredient to entering the Kingdom of Permanent Fat Removal," she says. "The act of *not* forgiving keeps us in the fat loop. But if we forgive our dietary transgression and move on, we are free of the inner tirade. And really, what was the crime? A piece of cake? One piece of cake does not a fat person make. All is forgiven. Move on."

Setbacks exist to teach you a lesson about where your inner strengths lie. If you give up on yourself because you ate a piece of cake, think about how and when you learned such values of defeatism. Where has giving up ever got you? See each setback as a lesson in self-acceptance and an act of forgiveness. Then, as Janice suggests, move on!

4. Super Support

It was when I was heading from a B to a D-cup bra that I realised this wasn't the kind of 'support' I had in mind. Good support is about having family and friends around you who aren't going to offer you cigarettes or cake (or whatever your poison) when they know you're giving them up in favour of new, healthier habits.

My husband, for example, wanted to be supportive of my decision to give up drinking wine on a daily basis, but still likes a drink himself in the evenings. So as not to put temptation in my way each evening by cracking open a bottle of wine to have with dinner, he now drinks beer instead. I'm not tempted to drink beer, so it's a good compromise and I'm appreciative of his support.

5. Keep Track

Keeping track isn't about the long and weary road you're trekking towards *goals*. Rather, this DIET defines 'keeping track' as celebrating your victories each day. Whether your victory is that you've had an alcohol-free day, or that you had a self-realisation, write them all down. These experiences make up the sum of your journey, and as you will realise when you see your journey on paper, happiness is a by-product.

You can keep track of your journey in a special journal, a plain old notepad or an online blog. It doesn't matter how you write it down, it only matters that you do.

This travelogue – the record of your journey – serves another purpose too. On days when you wake up feeling uggghhh, or when you succumb to an old habit, or you slip into an old self-criticism, you can read your journal and remind yourself how wonderful your life really is. Writing and reading about your blessings serves to remind you how lucky and brilliant you are. In other words, when you notice and acknowledge all the things you have to be grateful for, life responds in kind.

To illustrate this point, take my Daily Blissings gratitude project which entails taking a photo of something that I am grateful for each day. I upload each day's photo and comments to an online journal[3], and get enormous satisfaction seeing proof of my blessings right there on the screen.

As I say in my photo-blog profile, *"My mission: An exercise in gratitude by documenting a year of my life in photos – we have a thousand things a day that entertain us, inspire us, humble us and teach us, but there should be at*

*least one stand-out thing to be grateful for every day.
Taking a photograph of that 'thing' heightens
consciousness, increases intent and fills life with a sense of
purpose. Armed only with my camera phone and a budget
for MMSing one image per day, the challenge is not so
much about print-grade photos, but more about
consistency, resilience and dedication in carrying out this
mission of awareness."*

This Daily Blissings journal is just one way to keep track
of your journey. It *is* a challenge to keep the journal up to
date every day, but so rewarding. I totally recommend it.

In caring for your health there is no magical finish line
where you can throw your arms in the air in victory and
relax into a hot bath and a fluffy bathrobe. Of course, hot
baths and fluffy bathrobes are to be encouraged, but they
don't spell the end of the road for you and your journey
to well-being. So promise yourself that for the next three
weeks (even if you can't go on vacation), you will
consciously choose to step out of your old routine that
has you slaving to your old behaviours. Let little Johnny
make his own school lunches and car pool to school.
Allow hubby to hire a house cleaner to do your share of
the housework. Choose to delegate your work to your
staff and team mates. And clear your calendar of book
club, PTA, historical society or any other distracting
commitments. It's only for the next 21 days after all, a
mere blip on the timeline of your life.

What you do after the 21 days is up to you. But I'm
willing to bet that once you've broken these habits you'll
be wondering why the heck you should go back to them.
Leave old habits behind, along with your old baggage
(and lukewarm bottles of wine), I say.

Pssst. Remember: easy-peasy-orange-squeezy. Be *easy* on
yourself as you re-program your conditioned behaviours.

Reclaiming the Four-Letter Word

Yes, I've called this lifestyle concept and book *The Goddess DIET*, but I don't mean *diet* in the traditional sense of the word – that is, the penalty you pay for exceeding the feed limit. No, I mean to redefine this word so that it joins the ranks of *good* four-letter words.

The DIET I am talking about is *not* a punishment. It is *not* about starvation, regimen, sweat or sacrifice. This new DIET is an acronym for **D**aily **I**ntentional **E**mpowerment **T**ools. It is a reward for following a responsible, easy and holistic approach to good health and a glorious life. This holistic approach is made up of three essential facets:

1. **Your Body**

   The first part of this DIET is based on the single and simple principle of being kind to your body. Call it what you will – a vehicle, a temple, a house for your soul – in any case it needs maintenance to serve you well for the rest of your days.

   Your body is a barometer for your self-respect: disrespect your body and it will stop co-operating. You'll tire more easily, become grumpy more quickly, and get creaky when you move. Lord knows, a woman is only as young as her joints.

   How you treat your body is a direct measure of your self-worth. To improve your standing, this section focuses on increasing your awareness of how food and food types affect your body and health, and how the right combination of food and exercise makes you feel fabulous and comfortable in your skin. We'll also look at some easy ways to overcome toxic habits. With practice you'll be able to give your inner cynic the flick and give your body the respect it deserves.

2. **Your Mind**

Your mind and your attitude play a vital role in how you feel about your body and your life. This DIET dedicates a sizeable section to re-training your mind and your attitude so you can see good health is easy and achievable. It is also so you can see the exquisite beauty in your body and your lifestyle choices. Love your body, love your Self.

I will show you how to recognise signs of self-sabotage, and how to curb habits of self-criticism and self-destruction. This does take some commitment, but remember, it is simply conditioning that created the 'you' that you are now. And just as you were conditioned to be a certain way, you can certainly teach yourself to be another way.

3. **Your Spirit**

It is possible that as a child you were taught to rely on a greater power as your source of strength – Jesus, God/dess, Angels, Buddha, Shiva, the Universe, the Lord and Lady, a horny goat-god, an alien, Vogue magazine… There are as many faith systems as there are bubbles in my champagne glass. In this DIET, you are encouraged to reclaim your power from outer influences. To do this, there are various ways to take the responsibility for your self-love into your own hands. This way, you only have yourself to thank for your shining success ;-) We'll leave behind systems of deferred blame and gratitude, and empower ourselves instead by reconnecting with our authentic power within. I call this authentic power your 'inner goddess' – the beautiful and sacred being you were born to be. Love your body, love your Self, love your goddess within.

Now, I may be able to lead a horse to water, but it is *you* who must ultimately put the saddle on for the ride of your life. So aim to stay connected to your authentic power to maintain this DIET for happily ever after.

Let me put it another way… The Goddess DIET is intended to help you become passionate about:

- Doing right by your body so it can do right by you;
- Realigning your attitude for self-appreciation;
- Getting connected with your authentic power.

Three very easy principles, yes? The next step is to familiarise yourself with the three aspects of a successful DIET before you embark on your life-changing journey. It's easier than you think, especially as I'll be giving you a range of tools and tips to choose from. Please try them all at least once, then continue to work with those that resonate with you in the long-term.

Read the following three sections through once, without prejudice or expectation. Then read them again with a highlighter in hand. Circle bits that sing to you as these will most likely become the indispensable tools to help you succeed in your Diet.

1. **Body of Evidence** deals with food and fitness issues – love and respect the body you're in;

2. **Mind Over Matter** relates to how you see your Self – become aware of your values and your worth;

3. **Spiritual Enlightenment** examines your essence that makes it all possible.

You weren't born a wilting wallflower, a shrinking violet, or any other wimpy flower for that matter. You were born to be radiant. So open yourself to change and get your budding goddess positively blooming!

Body Of Evidence

My body is sacred,

a treasure and

a pleasure

A doctor on his morning walk, noticed an elderly lady sitting on her front step smoking a cigar. He walked up to her and said, "I couldn't help but notice how happy you look! What is your secret?"

"I smoke ten cigars a day," she said. "Before I go to bed, I smoke a nice big joint. Apart from that, I drink a whole bottle of whiskey every week, and eat only junk food. On weekends, I pop pills, get laid, and don't exercise at all."

"That is absolutely amazing! How old are you?"

"Thirty-four," she replied.

Why You Are 'Fat'

If you think you are fat, sadly there is no magic pill to get you to your ideal weight or size. It's completely up to you to change the way you treat your body so that it is as young, supple and beautiful as you want it to be.

Also believe that there is a real possibility that you're not really fat. (Or ugly, dull, lost, or whatever it is putting a lid on your radiance.) You only *think* you are. In which case you have been influenced by *perceived* expectations about what a woman should look like. According to the Better Health Channel[4] (a health and medical information service quality assured by the Victorian government), nearly half of all normal weight women overestimate their actual size and shape, and only one in five women are satisfied with their body weight. Furthermore, approximately nine out of 10 young Australian women have dieted at least once in their lives, and not always because health is an objective.

Negative body image is formed over a lifetime from many different influences including family, peers, media and social pressures. Think back to when you were a teenager and it was 'in' with your school friends to smoke a cigarette for lunch to save on calories. (Or was that just me?) Or when you were a rebelling young adult and dinner was a cask of wine and a handful of laxative chasers. (Oh please, that wasn't just me?)

A distorted body image (such as seeing a fat person in the mirror when in reality you're healthy) can lead to self-destructive behaviour such as a slimming disorder (anorexia or bulimia), dangerous dieting, or the disturbing Japanese trend to wrap oneself in cling wrap while singing karaoke. (Apparently singing one song while wrapped is the same as jogging 100 metres.)

One of your secret weapons in fighting negative self-image messages is your attitude. Understand that your body is sacred, a pleasure and a treasure. Be proud of your tummy that is feminine and round; walk tall like the warrior queen that you are, and wear your clothes as if you are a glamour puss (which, as you know, you are). It may help you to say this statement every morning during your 21-day transformation:

My body is sacred, a pleasure and a treasure

Another weapon is your understanding *why* you self-sabotage any efforts at getting fit, eating healthy food and seeing perfection when you look in the mirror. So, approach The Goddess DIET *not* with the notion that you will lose weight (although you probably will), but with the intention that you will a) lose conditioned and distorted thinking about your body, c) gain some tools to combat self-sabotage, and c) get a dose of good old-fashioned self-appreciation.

Before we deal with that though, let's be very responsible and define "how fat is *fat*?"

How Fat Is 'Fat' Anyway?

The most common method for measuring fat is the Body Mass Index (BMI). Whilst there are some short-comings in this method, at this stage the BMI scale is the most widely used way to determine when extra kilos could represent health risks.

Basically, the formula is used to estimate the relationship between your height and weight. A healthy BMI for an adult is between 20 and 25. There is a very easy calculator for determining your BMI at the Better Health Channel[5] website, but if you are virtually challenged, the simple formula for working out your BMI is:

$$\frac{\text{your weight in kg}}{(\text{your height in metres})^2}$$

Therefore, if you are 70kg and 159cm tall (as I was in the 'Before' photo), the calculation would look like this:

$$\frac{70}{1.59^2} \quad (\text{looks like}) \quad \frac{70}{2.53}$$

I had a BMI of 27.7, a result slightly over the healthy BMI range for an adult. Not too bad – nothing that an Attitude adjustment and a change in my lifestyle couldn't fix.

What BMI are you, and where do you fit?

- Under 18: You are very underweight and possibly malnourished. Please don't walk over any cattle grids without skis on. Gain weight now!

- Under 20: You are underweight and could benefit from gaining some padding.

- 20 – 25: You have a healthy weight range for young and middle-aged adults.

- 23 – 28: A healthy weight range for older adults.

- 26 – 30: You are mildly overweight, but ripe to become a Botticelli muse.

- Over 30: You are overweight or obese. If you have a waist size of over 35 inches (89cm) for women, you are at especially high risk for health problems.

Personally, I prefer to measure my 'fat' levels by the way my clothes fit me. My body has a natural weight where it likes to sit, and I know I'm at this point if my jeans fit me beautifully. Let's call this method the 'Jeans Test'.

So Do I Need The Goddess DIET?

Whether you need The Goddess DIET or not depends on your 'fat' test. This may have been achieved via your Body Mass Index results, or via your Jeans Test. Make sure you have conducted a benchmark test using either method before reading on...

1. You're **below** the ideal BMI or your jeans are loose. If this is the case, you're not fat. You only think you are. In fact, you are underweight and could do with a dose of good old-fashioned reality check. **Yes**, you need The Goddess DIET.

2. You're **within the ideal range** for a healthy BMI or your jeans look *hot*! If this is the case, you're not fat. You only think you are. Again, changing your perception about the padding around your middle will do you the world of good. **Yes**, you need The Goddess DIET.

3. You're **above** the ideal BMI or someone has moved the button on your jeans. If this is the case, it's likely you are a little (or a lot) 'fat'. Whether by a margin or a mile, learning good habits is going to do you good. So **yes**, you need The Goddess DIET.

OK, we've established that no matter what your size, shape or head-space, you need The Goddess DIET.

Whether it's to fix your perception of your body image, gain new and healthier lifestyle habits, or finding that limitless energy source to power you through life (or all three!), The Goddess DIET has advice to change your life for the better, for ever.

Bring on the goddess in the mirror!

How Crash Dieting Helps

How Crash Dieting Helps? Are you serious? The only reason I called this section *How Crash Dieting Helps* is to flush out the cheaters who skipped straight to this page! (Who wants to hear that achieving body-love takes time, willpower and effort, right?) This section also attracts those types who think a magic wand is still an option for achieving a body like Kate Moss. Or at least good health. One or the other. Can't say I blame you – I think we've *all* tried crash dieting at some stage...

So anyway, the bad news is that crash dieting is for suckers. The good news is that if you've done it, you're not alone. Most women have tried crash dieting at least once. It may have been that you starved yourself, taken laxatives, buzz cut your hair, hacked your nails to the quick and exhaled as you stepped onto the scales. How heartbreaking to find that you still weighed something!

Who can deny that the thought of going beyond skin-deep beauty didn't appeal at some stage? I mean, who needs two kidneys anyway? But enough of that. We're adults now. Now that we're grown up we need to be more sensible about things. And I mean *proper* sensible. Not 70s-style-mother sensible. Remember the fads they went through to lose weight? Like standing in a belt sander machine that sent wobbly bits into overdrive and martinis into orbit. No, we're not repeating our mothers' efforts or mistakes.

I'm talking about developing a rational and measured approach to healthy attitudes towards your diet, health, lifestyle and body-image. Something that is actually very easy to do. Read on... (or go back to the beginning if this section was the first page in the book you turned to!) ... and begin your DIET with these 21 Empowerment Tools.

21 Empowerment Tools For Your Body

This DIET is very easy, adaptable, forgiving and fun. You can experiment with as many or as few of the tools as you like, but like anything, you'll get out of it what you put in so do try to incorporate each tool at least once.

As it takes 21 days to revise or create a new habit, there are 21 tools to mix and match. Applying yourself to new practices will really help you smash any old habits, so do immerse yourself into each tool as you incorporate it.

Although you will naturally gravitate to the ones that will suit your lifestyle, at least familiarise yourself with all of the tools before you embark on your three-week holiday from routine. Once on your journey, be realistic about what you can or can't do depending on your agenda. For example, if you're going on vacation and flying for 16 hours, it will be pretty tricky to implement the Daylight Savings Rule, but you could find it a fun challenge to do the Brad Pitt Rule instead.

Record which tool you are implementing each day in your journal. At the end of your day describe how you applied the tool so that it worked for you. Tick off each tool from the Checklist as you use it so that you don't lose track or forget to use one of the tools.

Once you have tried all the tools during your 21-day journey, aim to incorporate at least three of them (or more) into your regular routine to appreciate your body every single day.

The tools form an acronym for *Healthy Life Robust Body*, which is beyond ironic – it's what you'll get when you apply them.

1.   Hara Hachi Bu

Hara hachi bu is a Japanese expression translating to "my gut is 80 percent full." It originated in Okinawa where the island inhabitants ate until they were only 80 percent full, which became a cultural habit of calorie control.

Combined with a plant-based diet with plenty of fish and soy foods, the moderate eating plan of *hara hachi bu* is thought to be the reason Okinawans register 80 percent less heart disease than citizens in the United States[6].

Stopping at 80 percent capacity makes sense, really. This is because your stomach's stretch receptors (the little messengers that send "I'm satisfied" signals to your brain) take around 20 minutes to register food filling it, and another 20 minutes after you've stopped eating to feel full.

The opposite of *hara hachi bu* is over-eating, or as the proverb goes, "digging your grave with your knife and fork." There are some easy ways you can avoid over-eating, such as:

- When dining out, order only an entrée (appetiser).
- Feed 20 percent of your meal to your dog before you start eating (make sure he doesn't develop a hierarchy disorder though!)
- Write down everything that goes into your mouth. It may be enough to make you conscious of eating with more moderation.
- Before you start eating, put some of your meal into a storage container for lunch the next day.
- Heed the words of American journalist, Robert Quillen, "Another good reducing exercise consists in placing both hands against the table edge and pushing back."

2.   Enter the Carb-Free Zone

Addicted to bread, pasta and hot chips? Join the club. My predilection for hot chips would explain the chestnut jelly in my thighs. Oh well, at least I enjoyed getting it there.

Breads and pastas are all foods that are loaded in carbohydrates (herein referred to as 'carbs') – one of the three food types that we rely on for specific nutrients. That is, we eat carbs for glucose, protein for amino acids and fats for fatty acids.

Carbs get a bit of a bad rap in that their role is to provide our bodies with energy in the form of sugar. Some diets espouse cutting out on carbs completely, but in my experience it's wiser to include a choice of complex carbs for balance. These are good carbs that are good for you.

As a general rule, 'white carbs' such as potatoes, white rice, white bread and white pasta provide us with *simple* carbs – the fast-burning form of sugar that fills us up quickly and gives us bursts of energy, but leaves us feeling hungry sooner. I always feel better, physically, by choosing 'brown carbs' (the good carbs) such as brown rice and whole grain breads and pastas. These provide *complex* sugars which are broken down over a longer period of time. This slow burn gives us more even energy levels and keeps a constant flow of serotonin (a feel-good hormone) flowing through our bodies.

Here are some tips to ensure you're eating the right carbs:

- When visiting your local sandwich bar, at the very least go for a nutty wholegrain bread, or order just the fillings without the bread. (This confuses the heck out of some staff, but do persevere!)
- The word 'whole' should be up-front in 'brown' products. This tells you all three parts (bran, germ

and endo-sperm) are present. Choose brown rice, wild rice, whole-wheat couscous, whole oats, whole rye and pop-corn. (*Pssst*. Brown rice absorbs toxins from the digestive tract helping to eliminate them from your body – double bonus.)

- At snack time, choose low-fat popcorn (a whole grain), or baked corn chips with Salsa (the chopped tomato counts as part of your daily vegetable intake.)

- Steer clear of energy bars and drinks. 'Energy' in this case means it contains a loading of simple carbs, which translates to nutritionally worthless calories.

- Be turned off junk snacks by this story about potato crisps. A report by the Department of Chemical Engineering at the Jordan University of Science and Technology[7] says that sodium acetate (the ingredient that helps give salt-n-vinegar chips that tangy flavour) is in trial to be used as an environmentally friendly concrete sealant. What the…?

A Word on Wheat

As an aside, wheat is a particularly tricky food in the carb group for as many as one in ten people[8]. It contains a protein called gluten that is a common food allergen. For many people it is difficult for the digestive system to break gluten down which results in fatigue, bloating and inhibited absorption of other vital nutrients. Simply by cutting wheat out of your diet is one way to eliminate bloating and allow your food to be digested properly.

Before I gave up wheat, I made several visits to three different doctors about my lethargy and weight gain – enforced napping after each meal was not how I wanted to live life. I got dozens of blood tests for conditions ranging from diabetes to gall stones, but the root cause of my downturn remained elusive.

On a tip from a friend, I gave up wheat – not an easy task at first. You'd be surprised at how many foods, particularly processed foods, contain wheat, so this took some research to get right. But I plugged away and within three days (yes, that soon!) it was as though a curtain lifted from my foggy brain. I ceased being so bloated, appeared as though I'd lost five kilograms, and I stopped feeling like I was walking through molasses. Suddenly I understood the cliché, "finding a new lease on life," because I was living it!

Ways you can reduce gluten in your daily diet include:

- Substitute traditional bread for bread made with spelt flour (a grain with very low gluten levels), or try breads, energy bars and breakfast cereals made with rice, millet, and other wheat-replacement flours.
- Choose crackers for your cheese that are made from rice, and that are baked (not fried).
- Make pancakes with buckwheat (it has no gluten) and use mashed banana or stewed apples or pears in the mix instead of sugar. I've also found a spot of almond meal adds an interesting texture and flavour.
- Many food manufacturers now make gluten-free alternatives for their range. You can find gluten-free pastas, crackers, breads, sauces and even muesli bars in the health aisle at your supermarket.

The Coeliac Society of Australia has been instrumental in influencing food labelling standards and supporting research regarding Coeliac Disease, Dermatitis Herpetiformis, the gluten free diet and any associated conditions. They have a resource-rich website where you can find diet advice and support groups at coeliac.org.au

3. Abstain After Six

I could never really understand how my Nana could be satisfied with a piece of toast and a cup of tea for her modest evening meal at the early hour of 5pm. But her simple habit turns out to grounded in good sense. That she is 99 years old and still living independently was proof enough for me, so I tried out her eating plan.

As it turned out, I lost six kilograms over six weeks simply by finishing my last meal before 6pm. Ah, the magic of sixes – who said 6-6-6 was a bad thing? This weight-loss is attributable to three factors:

a) My body had more opportunity to digest the food before it went into slumber;

b) The longer the gap between your evening meal and the previous meal or snack, the larger your dinner is likely to be. So having your dinner earlier gives you the edge in that you won't be tempted to load your plate; and

c) You wake up hungrier and better prepared to tuck into a substantial breakfast the next morning, thereby giving your body plenty of fuel to burn.

I didn't miss out on any of my favourite foods (or drinks) – I just ate them earlier in the day while my body was actively burning the food in my gut. Eating the major portion of my daily calorie intake earlier did wonders for my metabolism and ability to trim back down to my body's natural comfort zone.

Possibly the hardest part about this rule is changing your perception of when is the 'right time' to eat. Don't think you need to gorge yourself and slam your cutlery down at the stroke of 6pm. Simply adjust your eating times so that your last meal starts at 5pm and you are sated by six.

If you do sneak over the cut-off time, just go to bed later. Oh I can hear the night-owls singing from here.

Once you have mastered your new time habits, the next challenge is getting through the entire evening without snacking. Food is often used as a relaxant or a distraction at the end of the day, so be prepared with these tips:

- Make sure your last meal is a well balanced, high-fibre meal made up of the three main constituents (more on this in the Burnout Buster tool in this book).

- Brush your teeth after dinner. Brush them again if the snack cupboard beckons.

- Enjoy a cup of herbal tea in the evenings to keep your belly feeling full.

- Avoid boredom – this is a major reason why people snack. Find a hobby or an activity to replace your danger (time) zone of snacking. If TV is your habit, do something to occupy your hands – knitting (it's trendy again!), ride an exercise bike, cross-stitch, fold the ironing... (ha ha, I was just joking about that last one – if you're like me, you don't own an iron).

- If you're really struggling with not opening the freezer during the evening, apply the **30-Second Rule** by closing the freezer door and walking away to do a quick job to take your mind off it. Check your text messages, make a phone call, go to the loo.

 If you venture past the kitchen again and you remember the ice-cream, apply this principle again. Brush your hair, trim your toe-nails, drink some water, do some lunges right out the kitchen door...

- If you really really really must snack, opt for a tasty, crunchy, healthy snack such as the chick pea mix described in the Yummy Scrummy Mummy Love tool in this section.

4. Lubricate It

According to a women's gossip magazine, Catherine Zeta-Jones lost her baby weight by drinking lots of water every day. And I mean LOTS. Her rule of thumb was 30mL of water for every 500 grams of body weight.

Now, call her crazy (and I did when I tried this at home), but this ratio is insane. When I calculated how much water I would be drinking under C-Zed-J's reported plan, I came up with 10.5 litres. Around half of that certainly came right back up out of me when I attempted it.

But I'm sure the poor girl had the right idea at heart: Drink lots of water to flush toxins, hydrate the body and look cool at the gym. Water also flushes toxins from your vital organs, carries nutrients to your cells, moistens ear, nose, throat and eye tissues, and – here's the clincher – plumps out your wrinkles to help you look younger.

I'm sure it's no news flash to you that water makes up an enormous amount of our bodies: 82 percent of blood, 75 percent of muscle, 25 percent of bone, 76 percent of brain tissue, 90 percent of lung tissue, and 100 percent of my belly when I tried Catherine's plan.

It is generally accepted that eight glasses (two litres) of water a day is the ideal amount to keep you adequately hydrated, although a multitude of studies have proved varying suggestions over the years. Though no single formula fits everyone, knowing more about your body's need for fluids will help you estimate how much water to drink each day. I don't buy into the arguments – I just know what is right by my body by the condition of my skin (a longer term sign of success), how alert I'm feeling and, (an easy method), by the colour of my urine. It only takes a quick glance to gauge whether you're hydrated or dehydrated – your wee should be the colour of light

straw. If it is dark yellow or gold, you are dehydrated.
Use this little ditty to remember the rule:

> *If the wee is clear, never fear*
> *If it's the colour of straw, drink some more*
> *But if it's the colour of gold, drink three-fold*

Your water needs depend on many factors such as
existing health conditions, where you live and how active
you are. Whether you are a light exerciser or an extreme
workout kind of a girl, you can lose between two to a
whopping seven litres of water per day through sweat,
breath and urine. So, drink plenty of water throughout
your workout routine (in addition to your daily eight-
glass target).

In one of my empowerment stories for women,
BOTIBOTO, Beautiful on the Inside Beautiful on the Outside,
I listed some very easy ways to ensure you get eight
glasses of water intake per day. Try these ways to super-
hydrate yourself effortlessly:

- A glass upon rising;
- A glass at breakfast;
- A glass before leaving the house for work;
- A glass upon arriving at work;
- A glass at morning tea;
- A glass at lunchtime;
- A small bottle of water to sip at the red traffic lights
  on the way home; and
- A glass while preparing dinner.

Pssst. For an alternative to drinking water, try snacking
on watermelon, tomatoes and cucumbers — these are
between 90 – 95 percent water by weight.

5. Twice As Nice

Remember having endless energy to jump off bridges into a river? How about skipping rope with friends, building forts and cubbies all day long or climbing trees to chuck honky-nuts at your annoying little brothers?

Ahhhh, those were the days. Scabs on knees were a minor consideration compared with the thrill of splashing down, flying the cubby's new flag or having a honky-nut hit its target.

As adults, energies ebb and flow – there is no avoiding this. Some days we wake up ready to trek Nepal (or at least Chapel Street, Melbourne) while others it takes everything you have just to get dressed.

There is no doubt that during your 21-day process, you'll have at least one day of incredible energy. The sky will seem bluer, your partner sexier and with any luck, you'll actually want to play on the swings with your children.

Without delay, dilly-dallying or denial, make this your Double-It Day. Double the exercise, double the willpower, double the distance, double the fun.

Energy begets energy, so walk twice as fast, swing your arms twofold, and burn double the calories with everything you do.

Just *do not* double the food or alcohol – the ratio of food-in-sweat-out doesn't rise in proportionate measure. Besides, you do only have 24 hours in a day to work everything off.

Make this your affirmation today:

The more I move the more energy I have.

6.   Halvies Heaven

Recently I had a crowd over for dinner. In my poky little kitchen with limited pots, I was ill-equipped to prepare a huge meal. Put it this way: I gained a first-hand insight into how Jesus would have felt when faced with feeding 5000 people with just a handful of loaves and fishes.

But, my energies would have been wasted in stressing about something that can't be changed. Like the Dalai Lama said during his visit to Perth in 2007, "If you *can* solve the problem, there's no point in worrying about it. If you *can't* solve the problem, there's no point in worrying about it."

So, I just cooked up a huge bowl of (gluten-free) pasta and served up a small plateful to everyone – each plate ended up being around half of what I normally would have served. I told the crowd, "this is just an appetiser – part two is coming," then turned around and began cooking the second half of the meal.

Twenty minutes later the next stage was ready and I brought the platter to the table. Out of the dozen or so people that were around the table, only two people went back for seconds. The other 10 people declined a further helping, even though they would have eaten more had it been served up to them the first time around.

That's 83 percent of people that stopped eating because their stomach stretch detectors had registered they were full, and the interval between servings was sufficient time for my guests to realise they'd had enough.

I practised this concept during my vacation to Tasmania by asking the waiter at a restaurant to put half of my meal into a doggy bag for me to take home. Out of sight, out of mind, I didn't miss the other half of the meal when the plate was put in front of me. In fact, I was very satisfied with the half that I did eat that evening. Rather than finishing the meal by rubbing my belly and saying "oomph" (as I would have done had I eaten the whole lot), I had enough zing to suggest that we all walk back to the hotel rather than catch a cab.

Here are some other ways you can apply the Halvies tool into your diet:

- Split a main meal with your dining partner (or ask the waiter to doggy-bag half if you don't have a companion).

- Take the top layer of bread off your sandwich before you eat it.

- Halve your simple carb intake by choosing 'whole' options – wholegrain rice and bread, for example.

- Cut a pizza into 16 slices instead of eight. If you normally eat three slices, make sure you still only eat three slices.

- Halve the amount of alcohol you drink by replacing every second glass with a glass of sparkling water. Even if you end up drinking the same amount but over a longer period, at least you're re-hydrating as you're dehydrating.

- Buying food in bulk is healthy for the hip-pocket, but deadly for the hips. If you go to the movies and buy a large bucket of popcorn, for example, you're more likely to eat the whole lot. Buy a small bucket (if you must) and feel just as sated at the end of it.

- Halve your grocery bill: leave the processed meals on the shelf and chop up fresh vegetables instead.

7.   Yummy Scrummy Mummy Love

Remember when you were sick as a little girl and your
mum would bring you comfort food? Mine brought me
flat lemonade… which wasn't so great, but because we
were *never* allowed to have soft drink, even flat lemonade
was a treat. Nowadays, I'm pretty sure that medicating a
sick little girl with flat lemonade is accepted as an old
wives' tale. It didn't matter to me then though, and it still
doesn't matter to me now – as an adult I still think about
flat lemonade because it represents compassion.

Well, I *used* to… As part of The Goddess DIET I retrained
my natural attraction to this particular comfort food to a
healthier option. Now if I'm bedridden I drink a Vitamin
C loaded medicated drink instead, yet allow myself to
think that this was what my mother always gave me as
her way of showing me some mama-love.

In a report in Science Daily[9], researchers at the University
of California in San Francisco have identified a bio-
chemical feedback system (albeit in rats) that could
explain why some people crave comfort foods when they
are chronically stressed. The findings focus on a
glucocorticoid steroid hormone (corticosterone in rats,
cortisol in humans, but let's call it 'the stress hormone')
that prompts rats to engage in pleasure-seeking
behaviours in response to stress. Such behaviours include
eating high-sugar and high-fat foods, which subsequently
results in abdominal obesity. Or, in layman words: rats
got stressed, chose junk food, got fat.

Now, research also shows that terminal cancer kills rats
(who funded *that* research???), but I'm still happy to
acknowledge this study's assumption that comfort food
dampens the edge of chronic stress and hence, whenever
we get sick, anxious, depressed or cut off in traffic, we
reach for our favourite comfort food. It is easy to assume

that comfort food is high-sucrose (think, chocolate bars, tubs of ice-cream or flat lemonade) or high-lard (spicy chicken wings, fries and dim sims). I'm proposing, however, that there is a way to have your comfort food and eat it too, sans the caloric load.

Through personal experience I can tell you it is entirely possible to retrain your mind into eating a healthier version of your traditional comfort food, and still stimulate the appropriate neuro-chemicals that activate regions of the brain that stimulate pleasure. Sounds tiresome but it's really quite simple.

Here are some tricks to replace these tried-and-true comfort foods:

- Mashed Potato: Replace the lashings of butter or sour cream with fat-free chicken broth or crushed garlic. If you're serious about increasing nutrients where you can, replace 'white' potatoes with sweet potatoes for their carotenoids, a heart-protecting micronutrient.

- Gravy: Blend some chicken broth (there are some fantastic gluten-free stocks available now) with Worcestershire sauce and sliced mushrooms. For gluten-free gravy, thicken it with pure cornflour (although it's just as tasty in its runny form).

- Tacos: Give the saturated fat-loaded mincemeat a rest. Use premium mince or Textured Vegetable Protein instead. Once you've mixed TVP with chilli it tastes very similar to what you're used to. Hint: pretend you've never had a Taco and this TVP-style Taco will become your benchmark for flavour and texture.

- Fries: Lightly coat wedges of potatoes in grapeseed oil (this type retains its 'friendly fat' properties when heated to high temperatures), lay them out on an oven tray and bake them for 35 minutes at 250°C.

- 'Deep-Fried' Chicken: Remove the skin from your chicken pieces and brush them with peanut oil – another heart-healthy oil rich in monounsaturated fat. Roll the pieces in a combination of salt, paprika, ground white pepper and any other 'secret ingredients' you'd like to add, and bake for an hour.

- Chowder or cream-based pasta sauces: Replace the cream with low-fat evaporated milk. Creamed corn also makes a tasty substitute for thickened cream.

- Pizza: Make the crust from wholemeal flour. Substitute the bottled tomato paste with freshly sautéed cherry tomatoes, garlic and olive oil. Lose the fatty processed meats and use fresh ham or chicken breast. Add lashings of fresh vegetables. Replace the high-fat mozzarella with the lower-fat (note, low-*er*, not *low*, so still take it easy) grated edam or parmesan cheese or soft goat's cheese.

- Banana Split: Ditch the whipped cream altogether, halve your normal scoops of ice-cream, and puree a cup of fresh strawberries to replace the strawberry syrup topping. Sprinkle with 'LSA' (a mix of linseed, sunflower seeds and almonds) instead of peanuts.

- Peanuts: This chick pea mix satisfies the crunch and savoury burst you're seeking, but a with healthier choice of fats. Not only is it a yummy snack, but it will have your Italian friends in raptures with the memories it will evoke for them… Toss pre-soaked chick peas in a lightly oiled skillet until they begin to brown, then bake at 200°C for 20 minutes. Return the peas to the skillet with pepitas (pumpkin seeds), sunflower seeds and roasted slivered almonds. Drizzle the blend with a mix of 2 tablespoons each of honey and Worcestershire sauce, 1 teaspoon garlic powder and a dash of chilli powder. Bake again for 10 to 15 minutes, shaking the tray occasionally. Yum!

8.   Lighten Up

A friend once ate doughnuts as part of her diet regime. Her argument was that they were healthier than a slice of cake as there were no calories in the doughnut hole.

"Wow," I'd say, "you've saved upwards of three to five calories per piece of cake by doing this." The concept that by eating ten doughnuts she'd save 50 calories was lost on her, but we did have fun looking for other ways to eat treats with zero-calorie zones – the pockets of air in Aero bars, the CO_2 bubbles of gas in soft drink, the airy gaps in sponge cake, round biscuits (there are calories in the corners of square ones), and the cavernous holes in profiteroles that remain after sucking the custard and cream out. In these cases, the food simply acted as the wrapping for the low-calorie, low-fat serving of air. Gives a new meaning to 'empty calories', really.

Her rationalisation was a little flawed, but I did like the way that she looked for the positive in her eating habits rather than beating herself up for succumbing to a craving for a sweet treat.

Sometimes it's the guilt about what we're eating that weighs us down, more than the caloric load. The good news is that more and more manufacturers are coming up with healthier versions of traditional treats, and more and more researchers are coming up with reasons why eating treats is good for us (with conditions, of course).

Let's take the case of chocolate. Yes, I'll have two cases please, especially during the PMT stage of my menstrual cycle, ha ha. Chocolate contains valuable antioxidants that reduce the effect of dangerous oxidants, otherwise known as free radicals. These are introduced to the body via exposure to pollution, alcohol, unhealthy foods, stress and cigarette smoke (amongst other things), and cause cell breakdown in your body. This damage makes you more susceptible to nasty diseases like… oh who can think about evil things when you're eating chocolate?

Chocolate has more antioxidants than red wine, blueberries or black tea, but before you reach for a block of it, researchers say it's the dark chocolate that is healthiest. For example, a 40g milk chocolate bar contains more than 300mg of polyphenols – compounds known to provide much of the flavour, colour, and taste to fruits, vegetables and seeds, with antioxidant, antibacterial, anti-inflammatory, and anti-allergenic properties. Dark chocolate has more than double that and cocoa powder has four times that. So yes, you can eat chocolate, but remember that all chocolate is notoriously high in calories and fat, so go with Miss Piggy on this and "never eat more than you can lift."

While we're on the subject of lightening up, manufacturers are also providing us with an abundance of low-fat options now – light sour cream, skim milk, reduced-fat cheeses, low-fat mayonnaise and dressings, reduced-fat sausages and mincemeat, less-fat bacon, and light or low-fat ice-cream and frozen yoghurt… Be conscious as you're reaching for these options in the supermarket, and **read the labels**.

Labels that claim 'lite' or 'light', for example, may be referring to the colour or taste of the product but might still be high in kilojoules and/or fat. '97% fat free' goodies may be low in fat but can be laden with salt, kilojoules and sugar (often labelled as fructose). Out of 150 cereal bars tested by Choice magazine, for example, only 13 were nutritionally sound – most were so loaded with fat and sugar you may as well have been eating a chocolate bar or packet of chips.

9.   In Your Own Good Time

In a society that has rapidly adopted ready-made meals, packet mixes, frozen dinners and take-away fast fixes, I predict many kids won't have any trouble reproducing mother's Apple Pie when they grow up: they'll simply take it out of the freezer and heat it up.

When I hear reports that kids don't know where milk comes from (beyond the supermarket shelf), there's a lot of merit in understanding how meals are made, where ingredients come from, and savouring the process of creating them as much as the process of devouring them. That means getting back to basics and making time for your food.

I've become a fan of slow cooked food ever since hearing about The Slow Food Organisation[10], a non-profit group founded in Italy to counteract fast food and fast life. Their goal is to inspire you to take interest in the food you eat, where it comes from, how it tastes and how our food choices affect the rest of the world. With over 80,000 members in more then 100 countries, the movement aims to "preserve cultural food practices, including plants and seeds, domestic animals and traditional farming within local bioregions."

Since adopting some of their philosophies, I make a real effort to a) sit down to eat and b) incorporate local produce into my meals. Sounds simple, but really, how often do you sit down and consciously consume a meal?

To support my point, think about how you eat during the day. Chances are that at least once in the past week you've grabbed a bite to eat at your desk. You've also snatched an easy-eat item and devoured it on the run. These habits and clichés didn't enter our vernacular by mistake – we know about this style of eating because it is so common. So, try sitting down to eat your food, with consciousness, and really *taste* what's going on in your mouth. It's a party in there, so have fun.

Slow food is less instant, based on nature, and allows you more time to appreciate and understand one of the most important things to keep you alive: food. Sadly, there are only a handful of slow food events that happen around Australia each year, but don't let that stop you implementing slow food practices into your lifestyle.

Here are some simple ways to start:

- Pick up a corn chip. Just one. Smell it. Look at both sides, as many times as you like. Take a small bite. Notice what it feels like in your mouth. *What does it taste like?* Cardboard? Salty? More-ish? When you slow down and concentrate on what you're eating, more often than not, just one is enough to satisfy a craving for a snack.

- Make eating a sociable affair (and not just because 'he who eats alone chokes alone', as the proverb goes). One of my pet peeves is silence at a dinner table. Sure it's a sign that the meal is being enjoyed, but I'd still prefer to be sociable. By placing your knife and fork down between each mouthful means a) you have ample time to chew and taste each mouthful, b) you have time for quality conversation and c) you will eat less food in the 20 minutes it takes for your stomach receptors to tell your brain you're full.

- Turn your radio off. Restaurants wanting a high table-turnover (a nice way of asking for customers who eat and run), they'll often play high-energy or fast-tempo music. The theory is that the faster the tune, that faster you'll pig out.

- Sit next to a slow eater so you can pace yourself. Or, eat with just a fork (American style), or chopsticks.

- Another peeve is watching people talk with their mouth full. This grosses me out so much I put my knife and fork down and wait until they've finished their meal so that I can enjoy mine in a civilised manner. I am then able to eat with more gratitude and consciousness instead of having anger as a companion.

- Bless your food. How fortunate that you did not have to tend a crop every day no matter what the weather, to have this food on your plate. How incredible that we can eat a great variety of foods grown on our doorstep and all across the country. Give thanks for the technologies and diligence of others that makes this food readily available... See how each plate of food is a blessing? Express your gratitude by placing your hand over your heart and relaxing your anxiety about your attitude to food. Promise your body that this food is for nourishment, not to fulfil an emotional hunger, and enjoy every morsel that you place into your mouth.

- Always leave something on your plate. In some households an empty plate is an invitation for a second serving. If you have a Mum whose catchcry is "Eat! Eat!" leave a little on your plate in order to avoid the "let me get you some seconds!" pressure.

Confucius said, "the way you cut your meat reflects the way you live." I don't normally associate meat with lifestyle, but this analogy reflects the butcher's art of dissecting a beast so that all of it can be used to its best potential. Ultimately, this parallel encourages us to reflect on how well we utilise the time and resources we are given with this life. Do not take anything for granted – your health, your family, your youth, your wisdom, your energy, your energy sources... be consciously grateful for your food, its origins and what it can do for you.

10. Friends With Fat

In Hollywood movies police fall into one of two groups:
good cop or bad cop. In my kitchen, it's the fats that are
divided into two groups: good fat, bad fat.

Good fat? Yes, hallelujah, not all fat is evil. When eaten in
moderation good fats help nutrient absorption and nerve
transmission. They also regulate cholesterol metabolism,
promote skin and hair health and maintain cell
membrane integrity. (Ha! I wish they did the ironing too!)
Over-indulge though, and you're dealing with heart
disease, certain types of cancer and developing the girth
of an adult Redwood tree, so like everything, keep it in
moderation.

Good fats are the naturally occurring fats that haven't
been tampered with. They haven't been corrupted by
high heat, refining, hydrogenation or other sorts of
processing. So bring on the fish, nuts, seeds, avocados
and butter! Yes, creamy, delicious butter. I've been a fan
of butter ever since seeing Peter Russell-Clarke milking a
plastic cow for plastic milk (for margarine of course) and
singing, "butter tastes better!" Now I'll forego a sandwich
if it doesn't have real butter on it. (There you go, another
weight regulation tip: stand up for your morals!)

High on the hit list, superstar fats such as the omega-3
fatty acids (found in fish), and omega-6 fatty acids (found
in evening primrose oil) have been used to treat
conditions from bipolar disorder to skin problems. The
villain of the piece is named Trans Fats. Trans fatty acids
are a result of the hydrogenation process of liquid oils –
they undergo this process to better withstand the food
production process. Rule of thumb: if it has been
modified for a long life on the shelf, it is destined for a
long life on your hips.

Good Fat	Bad Fat
Monounsaturated Fats lower total cholesterol and LDL cholesterol (the bad cholesterol) and increase the HDL cholesterol (the good cholesterol). Peanut, grapeseed, flaxseed, canola, sesame and olive oils are high in good fats.	Saturated Fats raise your blood cholesterol as well as LDL cholesterol (the bad cholesterol). 'Sat fats' are found in meat, dairy, eggs and seafood. Some plant foods (coconut, palm and palm kernel oils) are also high in 'sat fats'.
Polyunsaturated fats lower total cholesterol and LDL cholesterol. Seafood and corn, soy, safflower, fish and sunflower oils are high in polyunsaturated fats. Omega-3 fatty acids (from oily fish) belong to this group.	Trans Fats are the bad boy in town. They raise LDL cholesterol (the baddy) and lower HDL cholesterol (the goody). Found in fast foods, pre-packaged foods, microwave popcorn and some margarines, they are bad, bad, bad, bad, bad.

Now, before you run off and relish this permission to eat fat, be aware that fat still has the highest calorie content of the 'three Amigos' (see Tool 14: Burnout Buster) and takes the longest to burn. So, be clever about which fats you choose.

My Favourite Fats

- Flaxseed is high in fibre and full of full of omega-3 fatty acids. It needs to be milled or ground for the nutrients to be released, but it is easy to buy it in this form. A naturopath once put me on two tablespoons a day which was easy to achieve by sprinkling it on food or blending it with shakes and cereal.

- Other seeds that I incorporate daily include a tablespoon each of sesame seeds (or Tahini), sunflower seeds and pepitas (pumpkin seeds).

- Avocados enable the absorption of fat-soluble nutrients. Compared to other vegetables avocado has a relatively high fat and carb content but if you eat it in moderation (around two tablespoons a day) it's a great source of heart-healthy monounsaturated fat.

- Olives or olive oil (raw) are great for salads, as are salad dressings that use olive, canola or flaxseed oils as the base.

- Grapeseed oil is excellent for cooking with as it retains its monounsaturated form even when subjected to high heat. Other oils can partially hydrogenate when they're heated, putting them into the bad fat category.

- Salmon and other omega-3 rich fish lower your risk of heart disease. They may also soothe a savage beast... WHFoods.com reports that out of 3581 young urban adults researched, those with the highest intake of omega-3 fats had only a 10 percent likelihood of high hostility scores.

Some Plump Is Not So Bad

Now onto the issue of body fat, Bruce M. Spiegelman of the Dana-Farber Cancer Institute[11] told *The New York Times*, "If you had no fat cells... you'd still be out of energy balance, and you'd put the excess energy somewhere else."

In other words, if you don't have any fat to store your excess energy, the energy is sent to your liver, which in turn can result in damage. (As if all that alcohol isn't taking enough of a toll!)

A reminder on healthy body levels: Be aware that 12 percent of a healthy woman's body is made up of essential fat to regulate your body temperature and cushion your organs and tissues, and body fat levels should range between 25–30 percent. (Remember the Body Mass Index test?)

If you've got a little padding around the waist, don't worry. This is *normal* and *healthy*. But if you're worried about a little roll, a few extra sit-ups each day may help. Also increase your water intake to help flush toxins and bloating, and practice the Brad Pitt rule (Tool 13) whenever you can.

The Truth About Eating Fat and Heart Attacks
(An oldie but a goodie)

* ❖ The Japanese eat very little fat and suffer fewer heart attacks than the British or Americans.

* ❖ The French eat a lot of fat and also suffer fewer heart attacks than the British or Americans.

* ❖ The Japanese drink very little red wine and suffer fewer heart attacks than the British or Americans.

* ❖ The Italians drink excessive amounts of red wine and also suffer fewer heart attacks than the British or Americans.

* ❖ The Germans drink a lot of beers and eat lots of sausages and fats and suffer fewer heart attacks than the British or Americans.

Conclusion: Eat and drink what you like... Speaking English is apparently what kills you.

---

11.   Empty the Waist Basket

Your stomach is *not* a trash basket. Well it can be, actually and that's precisely the point. It becomes a 'waist basket' when you throw trash down your throat.

While I insist that you should never feel bad if you cheat on an eating plan, I do urge you to think twice about what you're putting into your belly on a regular basis. Treats are wonderful and should be encouraged, but too much treating becomes trashing.

Sometimes there's no helping the urge to pick out all the marshmallow from a block of Rocky Road, followed by the nuts, then the chocolate itself. It's not like this happens all the time, right? But if it's happening more than once a day, reassess where your line is between trash and treat. For me, eating a wheel of Brie cheese over a week is a 'treat'; any more than that it becomes 'trash'. I know this because my jeans button is only too happy to remind me when I've overfilled the waist basket.

There are a few ways you can move on from little faux pas. One trick is to add fibre to your diet. You could also drink more water. Another approach is to flush toxins from your system with a detox plan.

Detox and Cleanse

Ideally you'll spend a *minimum* of three days on a detox plan, but even if you can't, at least you can minimise any damage by cutting down on coffee, tea and alcohol. Note: if you're pregnant or unwell consult your GP for advice.

Here are some other ways to improve your success in bringing back your healthy glow:

- Got a party season ahead? Avoid temptation by postponing detox plans until after any major parties.

- Stock up on fruit, vegetables and herbal teas such as peppermint, camomile, ginger or green tea.

- Get yourself a jazzy water bottle and keep it attached to your hip. Having water on hand (and hip) makes it easy to increase your daily water intake to the magical two litre ideal.

- Breakfast may be half a grapefruit, an orange and a slice of watermelon. Lunch can be a salad with baby spinach and vegetables high in water content (think cucumber and tomato). Dress salads with olive oil. Go the brown rice for larger meals and load up the steamed vegetables.

Apart from detoxing or taking the 'wishful shrinking' approach – (eating the cake standing up because there are no calories that way) – some painless ways to empty your waist basket include:

- Fill it with fibre. Fibre reduces your hunger, helps colon function and eliminates toxic and other wastes. Here are some painless ways to add fibre to your day:

  - Add a tin of baked beans to tomato-based pasta sauces, stews and casseroles. Alternatively try chick peas, kidney beans or cooked lentils.

  - Add bran to meatloaf, biscuit and pancake mixes.

  - Sprinkle seeds over your meals before serving.

  - Spread sandwiches with olive oil-based hommus instead of butter.

- Remove temptation. Keep any fatty foods out of sight, or give your stash to the kids to hide from you. Store treats in ceramic or opaque jars, or better still, leave them out of your shopping trolley to start with.

- Imagine you have eaten the cake already, and let that be enough for you.

12.   Renounce Pain

What kind of masochist came up with the idea of 'no pain no gain?' Sheesh! Why does it have to be hard? Choose an exercise that suits your character, aptitude and fitness level, and you'll be able to do it for much longer. Your motivation to exercise will increase because you *want* to do it. I mean, forget slogging it out at an aerobics class if you are there to convert fats, sugars, and starches into cramps, pains and bellyaches. Where is the fun in that?

I recommend you go with the school of thought that everything wears out eventually so you may as well be kind to your knees, back and heart by doing what comes naturally to your body type. So if aerobics gets you high, by all means do it. But if you're dragging yourself to each class and counting calories with every knee-up, find something else to do that you will actually enjoy and stick with in the long-term.

There is a list of some holiday activities you can do, and how many calories you are likely to burn in the process, over the page. Or if you've chosen a resort as your vacation destination, you can refer to the **no pain, no pain** list of activities instead. You won't burn as much energy, but you can alleviate any self-trashing or guilt by exercising your Attitude (see the Mind Over Matter chapter) with affirmations and positive thinking.

And for some fun, I've included a section on your perfect workout style based on your Goddess Birth Sign.

Before you start The Goddess DIET, highlight which activities you'd like to do the most, then consciously schedule them in to your 21-day program.

Activities For the Active Vacation

Activity, Calories/hour*		Activity, Calories/hour*	
Sitting in the car	85	Jogging, 8kph	500
Budgeting (what?!)	90	Swimming fast	500+
Standing in queues	100	Running after kids	500+
Driving	110	Hiking	500+
Dancing in your seat	180	Step Aerobics	550+
Walking, 5kph	280	Rowing	550+
Tennis	350+	Power Walking	600+
Skating/blading	420+	Cycling fast	650
Shaking your booty	420+	Squash	650+
Cycling, easy does it	450+	Skipping with rope	700+

Activities For the Resort Vacation

Activity, Calories/hour*		Activity, Calories/hour*	
Sleeping	55	Walking Tour, slow	220
Getting a facial	55	Golf without buggy	240
Eating (inc cutlery lifts, elbow bends)	85	Cycling in front of the gym's TVs	450+
Knitting (really?)	85	Mosh-pitting	420+
Lazing by the pool	85	Jogging, 8kph	500
Riding a tour bus	100	Swimming fast	500+
Playing mahjong	110	Escaping crowds	?

* Approximate

Activities According to Your Goddess Birth Sign [12]

Birth Goddess	Areas of Strength	Ideal Activities
ATHENA Mar 21 – Apr 20	Born leaders, Athena women are fiery and competitive. They like to get things done, and still look for more with energy to burn.	Burn off steam with high cardio sports: mountain-biking or cross-country running. Cool a fiery nature with snow sports like skiing.
JUNO Apr 21 – May 21	Happiest in a comfortable home, Juno women need to get off the couch and head outside. Bring your playmate if s/he inspires you.	Follow your earth-element bent with yoga, Qi Gong, hiking, or gardening. Rock-climbing and Pilates will keep you grounded.
PERSEPHONE May 22 – Jun 21	Persephone girls need variety. They can spend days in their own world, but make up for it with bursts of energy and intense health kicks.	Persephone loves coming up for air. Try martial arts or trampolining. Keep it balanced between high and low impact to bring harmony.
DIANA Jun 22 – Jul 23	Diana rules over nature and freedom of spirit. She rejects routine, preferring to hunt in the forest with her loyal dogs.	Take up hiking or orienteering. Pick up Diana's bow and try archery, or her sword for a bout of fencing.

PELE
Jul 24 –
Aug 23

Volcano-goddess Pele gives her girls lots of passionate energy and fiery qualities. They love being the social butterfly and the life of the party.

Zealous and proud, you'll love sweating it out playing tennis, basketball or beach volleyball. Cool down with yoga or stretching.

HESTIA
Aug 24 –
Sep 23

Creatures of habit and common sense, Hestia girls like life to be organised. They prefer burning the home-fires rather than their calories.

Structured classes such as aerobics and Tai Chi keep Hestia's mind and body happy. Rock-climbing gives you a great mental challenge.

VENUS
Sep 24 –
Oct 23

Sociable and flirty, Venus gals have a healthy capacity for pleasure, divine decadence, romance and all things beautiful.

Glamour sports such as polo, skiing or gymnastics are your best bet. Revel in your playful, sensual side with hot salsa or pole dancing!

BAST
Oct 24 –
Nov 22

The Bast gal is playful, strong, speaks her mind, and shows abiding patience to achieve her goals. Intense energy results when things do not go her way.

Use the calming nature of swimming, yoga or Qi Gong to soothe emotional stress. Free-weights or racquet-ball will help you focus on matters at hand.

RHIANNON Nov 23 – Dec 21	Magical Welsh goddess of wisdom, Rhiannon offers her girls a love of adventure. They are always on the move, seeking new skills and experiences.	Get on Rhiannon's white mare and go horse-back riding. Try sports where you can see the horizon: cross-country skiing, jogging and cycling.
DEMETER Dec 22 – Jan 20	Great mother Demeter is the champion of causes. Her energy inspires her girls to stop at nothing to achieve their goals, even at the risk of burn-out.	Concentrate on earthy pursuits: orienteering, hiking or abseiling. Balance your energies with aqua aerobics or rowing. Know when enough is enough.
HATHOR Jan 21 – Feb 19	Hathor women don't like things to stay the same. They can reinvent themselves to keep their interest levels fresh and life full of inspiration.	Your natural curiosity and airy nature means you need to mix it up. Try beach volleyball, jazz ballet, roller blading or soccer.
OSHUN Feb 20 – Mar 20	This African orisha inspires universal love and sensuality. Her water element causes Oshun-gals' energy levels to ebb and flow.	Go scuba-diving, wind surfing or white-water rafting. Purge fluid retention with martial arts and pilates.

13.   Oooh La La, Brad Pitt is Coming!

I once thought I saw Brad Pitt at the Bunbury Race Track.
Turned out the doppelgänger was actually the
bookmaker. Funnily enough, the champagne I'd enjoyed
not only fooled my eyes, it fooled my tongue as well –
instead of asking the bookie for a trifecta I was asking
Brad Pitt for triplets.

For the record, I note here that I would never say no to
triplets with Brad, champagne or none. The trick is
getting him to give me more than a second glance. I have
a strategy for getting a second glance incidentally, which
conveniently takes five kilograms off my appearance too.

Imagine Brad is walking towards you now… what do
you instinctively do? That's right – I bet you're squaring
those shoulders, sucking in the tummy, tucking in your
pelvis and thrusting out 'the girls' for a bigger dose of
sunshine. As much as we all hate to admit it, mother was
right in nagging us to keep our shoulders back and walk
like we have two books on our heads. The straighter
posture of shoulders-back-tummy-in aligns the spine,
adds to your radiance, and takes kilos off your bodyline.
The secret to maintaining this beautiful posture lies
within finding your natural centre of gravity and
strengthening your core muscles to keep you there.

It's also good to focus on your posture because, as we'll
find out in Tool 18: Burn Baby Burn, good posture fires
your metabolism. Yeah baby! And the added advantage is
that by looking the world in the eye and meeting it head-
on, you are sending the message, "I am here!"

So, on your Brad Pitt day, be conscious of beautifying
your posture and poise all day long. As you sashay
around town, make this your affirmation: "I'm here and I
matter."

14. Burnout Buster (Extend Your Battery Life)

Have you noticed how so many things come in threes?

- Fork, knife, spoon*
- Mind, body, spirit
- Past, present, future
- Paper, scissors, rock
- Sun, moon and stars
- Shake, rattle and roll
- Lights, camera, action
- Blood, sweat and tears
- Maiden, Matron, Maven
- Animal, vegetable, mineral
- Small, Medium, Large (aka, Scrumptious, Magical and downright Lurrrrvable)

(Yada yada yada.) Now I want you to add another Rule of Threes to your daily routine: the three constituents of a good meal. Let's call them the Three Amigos for the sake of this exercise – these are the three friends that you *must* invite to every meal. The Three Amigos are:

1. Protein for animo acids;
2. Carbohydrates for glucose; and
3. Fat for fatty acids.

Make sure that each of these three Amigos are included in each of your meals. In doing so you'll achieve the perfect combination of food to provide you with evenly balanced energy (fewer insulin spikes), a feeling of being sated for longer, and feeling less fatigued during the day.

---

* Take it from someone who knows: do *not* let your son holler for a "fork'n'knife" in an Irish accent at restaurants.

1. First Amigo: Protein

Leucine, Methionine, Valine… no, not the names of Bob Geldof's children, but three of the essential amino acids we need to build and maintain bone structure, muscles, vital organs and connective tissue. These amino acids can't be manufactured by the body, and are used to produce other amino acids and proteins, and glucose for energy.

To estimate the ideal amount of protein humans should eat daily, I pulled out my trusty Wahlqvist[13] – a textbook dating back to my University days of studying nutrition, but still a valuable resource in this century nonetheless.

Professor Wahlqvist recommends a daily intake of 0.75g per kilogram for a sedentary individual[14]. For an inactive gal weighing 70kg, as I was at the start of this DIET, this meant 52.5g of protein. This equates to a steak around the size of the palm of my hand – a very small steak compared to what I'm used to eating. As it turns out, even a tin of tuna provides 80 percent of my daily requirement. Cheap date huh?! This also means that *in theory* if I were to forego meat I could source my daily protein from an egg (13 percent), 1 cup of cottage cheese (50 percent) and a variety of snacks such as low-fat yoghurt, cheese and nuts.

Always combine your protein with the other two Amigos: carbs and good fats for the most efficient energy burn.

Tip: Make protein your first mouthful at every meal. This sets the tone for how your body processes the contents of your belly and converts it to energy – carbs first will result in an insulin spike, while the energy from protein is steadier, helps satiety and burns more calories.

2. Second Amigo: Carbohydrates

Some diet plans (that shall remain nameless) espouse increasing protein intake and eliminating carbs from your diet to lose weight. I have tried this and simply ended up wanting to stick my head in a bucket of pasta and not come out until I'd eaten the lot. I learned that it's just not right to deprive your body of an essential Amigo.

I firmly believe your body has a natural, inbuilt measure for detecting what it needs and it sends its order for that food, sometimes via cravings. (We examine this further in Tool 16: Spice-It-Up.) In denying yourself carbs, you're setting yourself up for a binge to satisfy your body's deficiency. Keep it balanced, however, and you're golden. Research undertaken in 2005 at the University of Washington School of Medicine[15] found that increasing protein while maintaining carb intake helps you feel fuller for longer, lose weight and (initially) decreases your levels of the hunger hormone, ghrelin.

So you don't have to cut out carbs to lose weight. Just be smarter about the *types* of carbs you eat. Revise Tool 2: Enter the Carb Zone if you can't remember which carbs to choose, but here's a hint: they start with 'whole'…

What's the best time to burn the carbs? Whether you choose to do resistance training (carrying the dog) or a cardio workout (chasing the dog), exercising is only good for you if you do it. Therefore, the best time to exercise is the time that it fits into your schedule on a regular basis.

The second-best time is within an hour of a snack of 200 or fewer calories, or in the two-to-three-hour window following a larger meal. The third-best time? Any time!

---

3. Third Amigo: Fat

Good fats play a vital role in your daily diet. They provide more calories than protein and carbohydrates, burns slowly for longer energy, and helps to maintain a feeling of fullness for longer periods of time. For a list of the good fats, refer to Tool 10: Friends With Fat.

A research team at Indiana University[16] recommends offsetting arterial damage by taking a walk within an hour or two after a high-fat meal. The study "obviously shows exercise is very effective in counteracting that high-fat meal," says Janet P. Wallace, a professor of kinesiology and lead investigator for the study.

How to help the three Amigos do their job better

- Ditch dairy foods. Some people are straight-out allergic to lactose, the major sugar found in milk. Dairy products also contain a protein called casein that is difficult to digest, and milk has an amino acid called tryptophan that has a sedative effect. As a trial, eliminate it from your diet for a few days to see how it affects your moods and feeling of well-being. You can still source calcium via beans, peas, sesame and poppy seeds and green leafy vegetables.

- Cut out wheat: Whether you have an intolerance to gluten or not, (many people do but don't know it), eliminate wheat for a while. Allergens stress your adrenals, which triggers the output of anti-inflammatory hormones, which in turn weakens your adrenals over time. This increases your propensity to stress and can make you more vulnerable to fatigue and low energy.

- Reduce caffeine. The caffeine kick you get in your daily java could be doing you damage if you overdo it. Too much caffeine stresses the nervous system thereby *depleting* energy rather than *giving* you energy.

I mentioned earlier that I'm not recommending anything in this DIET that I haven't tried and tested myself. So yes, I cut down on my coffee intake and trust me, it doesn't hurt as much as you might think. Absolutely have your morning fix, (it does contain anti-oxidants, after all) but opt for herbal teas or decaf (aka the 'why bother' coffee but there *are* some good ones out there) and within a few days you'll be feeling less jittery, nervous and irritable.

Signs that you are drinking too much coffee:

❖ Your eyes stay open when you sneeze;

❖ You answer the door before anyone knocks;

❖ Instant coffee tastes good even after an instant;

❖ Your parking inspector gives you speeding tickets;

❖ There's a photo of your coffee mug on your desk;

❖ Walking 20km on a treadmill is not a problem, even if it is unplugged;

❖ It doesn't bother you when your coffee grinder breaks down because you can use your teeth;

❖ You'd breastfeed your baby but it would keep him up all night;

❖ You power nap often just so that you can wake up and smell the coffee; and

❖ You ride your exercise bike to work.

Mixing and Matching the Three Amigos

If you want to get into the nitty gritty of what's in your food choices, the United States Department of Agriculture[17] has a comprehensive online database of nutrient profiles for 13,000 foods. These are foods commonly eaten in the States – I know because I looked up 'cheese' and got 519 food codes, including the mind-boggling imitation aerated cheese in a can. Where else but America has such a variety of product on their super-market shelves?

But if you just want a simple rule of thumb to work with, use this one. When planning how to mix and match your three Amigos, imagine you are looking at a dinner plate. One quarter should be carbohydrate (rice or pasta for example), a quarter your meat or protein serving, and half should be vegetables or salad. Following are some ideas for how to mix and match your three Amigos at each meal. Note: choose only one protein type per meal.

Choices For Your Meal Plan

	Protein	Carbs	Good Fat
Breakfast	Egg(s), Bacon, Yoghurt	Fruits, Wholegrain toast	Sunflower seeds, grapeseed oil
Lunch	Tuna, Smoked salmon, Cheese	Salad, Crispbread, Whole bread, Rice crackers	Pepitas, Almonds, Avocado, Olive oil
Tea	Meat, Poultry, Fish	Vegetables, Brown rice, Rice noodles	Omega-3 in fish
Snacks	Green tea for its anti-oxidants		

The following combinations are examples of light meals that I enjoyed in the weeks following my vacation. It was incredible how I didn't feel hungry for the five hours in between each meal, and I didn't experience the 3 o'clock slump during this time. You will notice that because I'm on a gluten-free diet, these meals suit me. I planned them in advance so I had the gluten-free ingredients on hand, and I encourage you to do the same.

Vegetable Omelette

Whisk two eggs with some water, seasonings of your choice and a handful of finely chopped up vegetables – broccoli, mushrooms, baby spinach and capsicum is a tasty combo. Pour a drizzle of grapeseed or olive oil into a frying pan, then your egg mix. Cook on low heat until the top of the omelette begins to set. Fold in half and serve. Note: If possible, don't add cheese or milk as this is mixing up your protein types.

Fruit Yoghurt Smoothy

Blend together five tablespoons yoghurt, one diced green apple, a handful of flaxseed, five almonds, and your choice of another piece of fruit: kiwi, fresh strawberries or frozen berries. You might choose to avoid bananas because of their high Glycemic Index, but ask your body what it needs and act according to the answer. Pour the mix into a bowl and sprinkle with sunflower seeds.

Smoked Salmon (or Cheese) Crackers

Spread four gluten-free crispbreads with a quarter of a mashed avocado. Sprinkle with finely chopped sugar snap peas, red capsicum, almonds and sesame seeds. Lay no more than 20g of smoked salmon <u>or</u> low-fat cheese over each crispbread and garnish with a generous helping of sprouts. Note: Do not combine the salmon and cheese as this is mixing up your protein types.

Baked Ginger Fish and Vegetables

Whisk together grated fresh ginger, a crushed garlic clove, one tablespoon sweet chilli sauce and two tablespoons each of gluten-free soy sauce and mirin. Place a salmon steak in the centre of a piece of foil and spoon marinade over each steak. Top with thinly sliced shallots and a slice of lemon. Wrap the fish in the foil and place it on a baking tray in a pre-heated oven at 220°C and bake for 15 to 20 minutes.

While this is baking, steam some 1cm thick slices of butternut pumpkin for 10 minutes or so, and half a bunch of bok choy for five minutes. Alternatively, steam the vegetables of your choice, or go the Raw Food route with capsicum, carrots and sugar snap peas. To serve, remove the fish from the foil and place in a shallow bowl. Pour juices from the foil parcels over the top, and serve with the pumpkin and bok choy.

Fried Rice and Chicken

Wash a cup of wholemeal rice and simmer it in two cups of boiling water until al dente. Leave the rice to cool while you cut up a chicken breast (skin off) and a variety of vegetables such as shallots, broccoli, snow peas, zucchini, capsicum, corn kernels and so forth.

Lightly coat the bottom of a wok with grapeseed or olive oil and seal the chicken. Once it is browned, add the vegetables and stir-fry for a few minutes. Add the rice to the wok and toss all the ingredients until they are warmed through. Add chilli and herbs to suit and drizzle a measure of gluten-free soy sauce and mirin until the rice is lightly coated. Remove from heat and stir through roasted almond slivers. Serve with a sprinkling of sesame seeds and garnish with sprouts.

15. Upside Down and Inside Out

Remember my Nana from the Abstain After Six tool? Her evening meal could consist of tea and toast – what might be considered breakfast for some people. This got me to thinking – "what if I had a day where my evening meal was first, and my breakfast were at the end of the day?"

In theory, it would mean that the highest portion of my calorie intake would happen straight up. My body would have plenty of opportunity to burn this energy throughout the day, meaning less would end up on my spare tyre than had I eaten the same meal at night.

Another advantage is that I would feel super-sated, so I could gradually taper down my food intake at lunch and through to tea-time. This means less chance (and desire) for snacks to fuel sagging energy during the day, and my metabolism can work full-speed during my awake hours.

Win, win, win, win, win, win, win.

Now, I'm not saying breakfast should now consist of fatty meats, gravy, bread and lots of butter, roasted vegetables and ice-cream. But you could try opting for a big breakfast at the corner café, remembering to choose only one source of protein: eggs *or* bacon *or* cheese per Tool 14: Burnout Buster. Your metabolism will fire up with eyes wide open and, providing you don't graze on sugary snacks to produce insulin spikes, it will continue to burn evenly. In other words, choose to make breakfast your major meal for the day for energy to burn all day long.

Lunch can remain as normal, then taper down your food intake for a very light supper. If you do it right, a light evening meal will be all you're in the mood for anyway.

16. Spice-It-Up

I once had the privilege of meeting Don Tolman, a
campaigner for self-care and self-education and author of
The Farmacist Desk Reference (Benacquista Publishing
2007). He showed me something about food that
scientists now call Teleological Nutritional Targeting, and
that is, "Every whole food has a pattern that resembles a
body organ or physiological function."

Furthermore, this pattern can be interpreted for how that
food benefits you. Carrots, for example, when sliced look
like the human eye. Surprise surprise, Teleological
Nutritional Targeting confirms what every grandmother
has ever said – eat your carrots, they'll help you see.

The lesson in Tool 16 lies within Don's steadfast belief
that he intuited how his food affected his health. He
knew tomatoes were good for his heart before science
confirmed it to be true. He knew that women should eat
avocados before science confirmed that eating one a week
"balances hormones, sheds unwanted birth weight and
prevents cervical cancers.[18]" He knew all this, because he
listened to his body and acted upon the messages.

Such trust in your own body is a skill you'll need when
trying this Tool. There is so much conflicting evidence
about whether herbs and spices are beneficial to weight
regulation. Some say yes, others no… so, you decide.

Herbs and spices have been used for centuries, for many
reasons. European merchants paid port taxes using
'grains of paradise', Hippocrates suggested using garlic
to treat illness, certain spices are used to preserve meat,
and all of them are used to make food more interesting.
But lately it is fashionable to claim that certain herbs,
spices and even berries will help speed up your
metabolism, burn fat and assist with weight loss.

Let's look at chillies, for example. The theory goes that thermogenic herbs increase the body's temperature and blood circulation and in so doing, helps the body burn more calories. As researchers at the Institute of Food Technologists[19] observed, however, nearly 70 clinical studies on spices have yielded inconsistent results.

To add to the inconsistencies, the ABC's fabulous, crazy-fun and lovable science guru, Karl Kruszelnicki, says, "Eat chilli, eat more."[20] His theory is that chilli inhibits the nerves connected to your stomach stretch receptors thereby slowing messages to your brain that you are full. If your brain doesn't know you're full, you'll keep eating. I tested this once by adding extra jalapeño peppers to a pizza. I found his theory to be credible when I ate twice as much pizza as I normally would have, possibly due to numb taste buds. Or probably just because it was *tasty*.

So, take any un-referenced advice with a grain of salt (ha ha). Rely on good food and fitness habits to maintain your health, and if offered a miracle herb, listen to your body: do you need it?

As for good health, that's a different matter. Many herbs are known to have the double advantage of adding flavour to a meal *and* health benefits to your body.

- Ginger improves your mood and inhibits nausea;
- Cinnamon curbs exhaustion and lifts your mood;
- Peppermint and camomile soothe ratty nerves and help relieve tension;
- Garlic, turmeric and ginger add flavour, flush toxins, boost immunity, fight infections and alleviate aches;
- The humble basil helps clarify your mind, so a large batch of pesto at exam time could be good; and
- Fennel can be used to help with bloating, flatulence, mild digestive spasms, and coughs.

17. To Digest, Divine

I don't know what was happening in Mark Twain's life when he said "To eat is human, to digest, divine," but I suspect a good dose of fibre and a fix of digestive enzymes may have helped him out somewhat.

If you're living with bloating, flatulence, irregular bowel movements, cramping or excessive gurgling in the pipes, chances are you're one of the gadzillions of women who are likewise experiencing digestive dis-ease. There are things you can do improve your digestive health, and it's important that you do – if you're not digesting your food properly your body is missing out on the vitamins and minerals it needs to make digestive enzymes that break the food down in the first place. A vicious cycle. Here are some obvious tips for improving your digestive health:

- Eat 'whole', unrefined and unprocessed foods;
- Eat seeds, beans and legumes rich in digestive enzymes;
- Eat vegetables raw;
- Eat specially-fermented foods such as yoghurt enriched with acidophilus;
- Limit your intake of coffee and high-sugar drinks;
- Avoid heavy meals laden with starch and stodge;
- Eat foods that are rich in digestive enzymes such as melons, papayas, sesame seeds, oat bran and beans.

There are many types of enzymes that all specialise in breaking down separate components of the three Amigos. I could go on about the range from alpha amylase to the protease enzymes, but the real point is, if your discomfort persists, consider taking some enzyme supplements (available from health food stores).

18. Burn Baby Burn (Energy, that is)

There is a little coordination test that catches everyone
I've tested it on. It involves spinning your right foot
clockwise then drawing the number '6' in the air. Go on,
try it yourself. I'll give you half a second while you do…

Muzak, funky background muzak playing while you spin
and draw… Time's up… What happened?

Your foot started spinning ante-clockwise didn't it?! So
far I haven't met anyone yet whose foot doesn't
automatically stop spinning clockwise and starts going
in the other direction.

Anyhoo, the reason I'm talking about spinning ankles is
because it's a good, subtle and easy exercise to do while
you're sitting in a car or train. It tones the calf muscles,
aids circulation, increases your metabolism and helps
whittle down piano-legs.

Before I started The Goddess DIET, I preferred lie-downs
to sit-ups. Truth be known I still do prefer lie-downs, but
the incidental exercises like ankle-twirling mean at least
I'm doing *something* to increase the rate at which my body
burns the energy I've put into it.

Yes, even the act of preparing fresh food can count as
incidental exercise. Chopping, shredding, stirring and
rubbing your belly burns more calories than popping a
frozen meal into the microwave. In fact, a team led by
James Levine at the Endocrine Research Unit at the Mayo
Clinic in Rochester[21] found that people who fidget and sit
down less put on far less fat than the couch potatoes who
stay slumped in front of the TV or desk.

Levine et al. (1999)[22] overfed people and found that
putting on weight was directly affected by NEAT: Non-
Exercise Activity Thermogenesis – a term to describe "the

energy expended by physical activities other than planned exercise and includes fidgeting, standing, walking, and postural movements."

In a follow-up study Levine et al. (2005)[23] studied obese couch potatoes that remained seated for about 2.5 hours longer than a comparative group of lean couch potatoes. They estimated that the leaner sofa spuds burned up an additional 350 calories per day simply by fidgeting and getting off the couch more often.

The message here is, if you're a couch potato and intend to stay that way, at least twirl your ankles! Even the smallest difference in your energy balance can result in long-term weight gain or loss. Other than that, here are some other ways to incorporate NEAT into your day:

- Park the car a mile away;
- Mop the floor to salsa music;
- Run to the phone when it rings;
- Curl your biceps while on the telephone;
- Bounce on a fit-ball at your desk instead of sitting;
- If you have a chair, twirl: 60 twirls burns 50 calories;
- Jump up and down upon hearing exciting news;
- Do pelvic floor exercises while at the traffic lights;
- Strap on a pedometer and aim for 10,000 steps a day;
- Run to the gym (what you do once there is up to you);
- Do brief bouts of exercise (10 tummy tucks, 10 buttock clenches, 10 squats) as the kettle boils.

Neat huh? Even chewing gum burns 11 calories an hour, but the offset is that chewing makes you hungrier sooner, so choose your battles wisely.

Move It (Up a Notch)

There are two types of people in this world: those who
are born to exercise, and those that can't be bothered.
I used to be in the latter category. When I did decide to
exercise I made it early in the morning before my brain
could figure out what was happening. Upon awakening,
I would instruct myself, "Up. Down. Up. Down." Then,
after two strenuous minutes, I would move on to the next
exercise with, "OK, now the other eyelid."

To help the shift from "Good Lord, it's morning" to
"Good morning Lord!" be conscious that exercise is a
lifestyle change, not a weekend romp. So find something
you love doing and will want to do often. While on
vacation in Tasmania, for instance, I rediscovered my love
of walking, hiking and exploring my world on foot.
Likewise, if you love walking choose a holiday
destination that will give you lots of opportunity to hit
your stride – Cinque Terre in Italy, for example, or
walking cities such as Venice or Manhattan.

In Australia, national guidelines[24] recommend 2.5 hours
of moderate exercise a week – this works out to around
30 minutes a day. The United States Department of
Agriculture goes one step further and recommends
60 minutes a day to prevent weight gain, and up to 90
minutes to help with weight loss. Here are some unique
ways to exercise without the pain:

- Adding just 2000 more steps to your day can prevent
  weight gain, says Dr James Hill at the University of
  Colorado Health Sciences Center[25]. Walk your dog to
  the furthest tree for his wee, walk on the spot while
  watching TV, or pace while talking on the phone.

- Burn more fat on your treadmill by warming up, then
  setting the speed to a brisk jog for one minute. Reduce

the speed to a walk again, take a drink of water and walk for two minutes. Increase the speed again for one minute. Repeat this cycle for 10 minutes (or longer if you're comfortable) and you'll get a longer, easier workout than had you run flat-out from the start to the finish.

- In Tool 3: Abstain After Six, I mentioned a 30-Second Rule for distracting your mind from craving treats. There is another 30-Second Rule I'd like to introduce you to here. First up, find a golf course and play a round or two. If you tee-off badly, you have 30 seconds to retrieve your ball and have it back on the tee. If you can do that in less than 30-seconds your first swing doesn't count. This particular 30-Second Rule gives you another win-win: your waistline looks good with the extra running, and your scorecard looks good too.

- Encore! If you want a longer life, pretend you're the conductor of an orchestra. Their 'wing-flapping' motions give them an awesome cardiovascular workout.

- Become Sir Dance-a-Lot. How is it that James Brown didn't die at 27 like Jimi Hendrix, or at 21 like Sid Vicious? With his never-ending high-kicks, air-jumps, mid-air splits and energetic whoops into the mike, James did the equivalent of a step class at every performance.

At the risk of sounding like a broken record: To complement your efforts, drink green tea. It is thought the catechins in green tea protect a brain chemical related to metabolism. The higher your levels of this chemical, the faster your metabolism. Each cup of brewed green tea contains around 100mg of catechins – around three cups a day should do it.

Seeing Exercise and Food in Motion

Imagine your food intake and your exercise tally has to balance on your body's profit-and-loss sheet at the end of the day. Don't burst a blood vessel over this – I'm just using this to illustrate a point.

Remembering that > is the symbol for 'is greater than', here are some rules of thumb:

- Food In = Energy Out.
- Food In > Energy Out = Weight Gain.
- Energy Out > Food In = Trim Down Tone Up.

If it takes 116 minutes of walking to burn off a bucket of hot chips, for example, achieve a balance in Food In = Energy Out by finding a fast food joint that's a two-hour return journey on foot.

I can hear you gasping – *you expect me to walk for two hours for a lousy bucket of chips?!* Well, first off, I'm not expecting you to do anything – you are in charge of your own choices! Secondly, everything is in walking distance if you have the time. So assume walking is fun (which it is), and do it! With any luck, by the time you've arrived you'll only feel like water instead of hot chips – there's another win-win for ya!

For inspiration, consider this little poem by W.H. Davies.

> *Now shall I walk*
> *or shall I ride?*
> *"Ride," Pleasure said:*
> *"Walk," Joy replied.*

Also remember that the best remedy for a slow metabolism is a long walk – toning up and gaining a life is literally a walk in the park!

Walking For Weight Loss

Food	Quantity	Minutes walking*
Cup vegetables	1 cup	9 mins
Banana/apple	1 medium piece	25 mins
Pizza	1 slice	40 mins
Coke	375ml (large can)	41 mins
Potato Crisps	50g packet	68 mins
Mars bar	60g	72 mins
Sausages	150g	85 mins
Hot chips	225g (1 cup)	116 mins
Meat pie	1 individual	125 mins
Chocolate	100g	140+ mins
Chops	2	170+ mins

* 'Minutes of Walking' is based on a moderate pace that causes a slight, but not noticeable, increase in breathing. Here are some gauges for measuring your walking speed:

- If you can talk easily while walking, you could probably push up your walking speed a notch;
- If you can sing while you're walking, you're probably annoying your fellow walkers;
- If you can chew gum while walking, you're probably a great multi-tasker.

Pssst! Become a member at 10000steps.org.au and track how many steps you walk per day as motivation.

19. On the Wagon

If you're watching your waistline, alcohol is the perfect
tool for putting your spare tyre right out in front where
you can see it. Each gram of alcohol contains seven
calories per gram (150-200 calories per glass), compared
with the relatively restrained four calories per gram in
regular carbs. In other words, indulge in just three small
drinks and you've drunk the equivalent calories of an
entire meal.

Furthermore, alcohol turns off your fat-burning
hormones. So if you're seeking to *increase* your lean body
mass (that is, put on weight), drink at night when your
metabolism is at its slowest and your fat-burning
hormones have been put to sleep.

If it's true that most accidents happen at home, then
when it comes to alcohol I'm entrenched in a world-class
hazardous hot-spot. Living in Margaret River, the world's
premier wine region, has proved time and again to be a
residential hazard. How can one resist trying *all* the new
vintages of a favourite label after all? Or screwing the top
off a cheeky Sem Sauv Blanc as the little hand hits 5pm?

Yes, winding down with a glass of wine after work,
another glass while preparing dinner, another glass over
dinner... (do I dare say "etc"?) can be very habit-forming.

Going on vacation doesn't necessarily make it easier,
either. There are new labels to learn and love, new
wineries and breweries to explore, long lunches to laze
over and dining out is pretty much a given. Take comfort
though – it's a habit that's not impossible to break. Note
that for this Diet, I'm simply suggesting that you break
the *habit*, not your bottles.

Here are some tips for cutting down on your intake:

- Rather than 'drinking like a fish', drink what a fish actually drinks – water.

- Go on a *walking* winery tour and walk from winery to winery. Avoid walking through vineyards though – you might get yelled at for traipsing through the vines, (as happened to me once).

- Mix your drinks with soda water to rehydrate as you dehydrate. You'll drink less alcohol content.

- Learn from UK journalist Nicky Taylor's investigation into binge drinking[26]. She drank a staggering 516 units of alcohol over 30 days and aged 11 years.

- Do your exercise exchange (see below) before you drink. Exercise gets the endorphins pumping so you will feel less likely to want to numb the 'feel good' sensation in your body.

- Be conscious about why you're having another glass of wine, or why you're having the first glass at all. Ask yourself, "How is this wine enhancing my day?" and "Is it worth the exercise exchange to work it off?"

Exercise Exchange For a Glass of Booze

Exercise	Minutes Exchange (approx)		
	Beer, Stubby 138 cal	Spirits 30mL 105 cal	Red Wine 100mL 70 cal
Reading	70	50	35
Disco Dancing	26	20	13
Walking 5kph	20	15	10
Jogging 8kph	13	10	6
Breast Stroke	12	9	6

20.   Daylight Savings

God/dess bless Benjamin Franklin, I say. As a father of
Daylight Savings, he not only saved Paris thousands of
candles, but had them opening their bedroom shutters
well before noon. He also inspired this particular tool.

The Daylight Savings tool is one that I use from Spring
Equinox onwards (20-23 September in Australia.) At this
time the mornings are getting lighter earlier, so it's easier
to get out of bed. Furthermore, the weather is getting
warmer so I don't have to fight for beach-space with the
penguins and icebergs when I go walking.

I simply apply this rule by putting my bedroom clock
one-hour forward before I go to bed. Then I get up at my
normal time (around 7am), go for an hour-long walk, and
when I get back it is still magically 7am according to the
kitchen clock (even though it is 8am in my bedroom.) It is
a great way to squeeze an extra hour into every day
without having to get up any earlier.

It's also a good thing to make sure it's only your bedroom
clock that you change. This will also trick your mind into
thinking it's later than it really is when you go to bed so
that you're less tempted to read "just one more chapter" –
it is much healthier to catch some vital zeds instead.

Americans have a fabulous rhyme for remembering how
to handle your clocks for Daylight Savings:

> *Spring Forward,*
> *Fall* Back*

Pssst! You don't have to stop this rule in Autumn!

* 'Fall' is the American word for Autumn but it doesn't
really work for us to say "Autumn back", hence the
Americanism in this instance.

21. Yes, yes, yes, yes, yes, yes and yes

To eat a small meal now or a big one later, or both? That is the question. On one end of the scale, there are people like Jorge Cruise (*The 3-Hour Diet*) who recommends eating a small meal every three hours and stopping three hours before bedtime. On the other end of the scale, Gary Schwartz[27], a researcher with the Albert Einstein College of Medicine, says "there is no strong data supporting either ... as being more effective."

Personally, I do understand the concept that eating every three hours creates a nice ritual whereby meals can't be forgotten. From experience, I do tend to get absorbed in tasks at hand and accidentally skip meals during the day. Naturally this sends my metabolism plummeting and my Irish genes racing into famine mode. I know when I've been naughty when I can hear these survival genes screaming as they race around my body looting any glob of fat that was otherwise minding its own business. "Quick!" they yell as they stuff more fat into their hand baskets. "More fat for her ankles!"

All of this in scientific terms: ritualised eating increases your baseline metabolic rate which increases energy, decreases appetite and... meh, I like my explanation better. Besides, there are so many for-and-against arguments about whether we are metabolically better off eating three regular meals or six smaller ones, it gets bamboozling. I have tried the six-small-meals approach and personally it didn't suit me. But it *may* suit you, so dedicate one day during this Diet giving it a try. If it gets you eating healthy food instead of starving and bingeing, well then it's probably a good thing for you.

In short, let's boil this tool down to one simple factor: say **yes**. Say **yes** to breakfast, **yes** to a regular eating regime, **yes** to eating less calories overall, (whether it be by eating less food or eating less often), **yes** to burning more calories, **yes** to healthy snacks in between healthy meals and **yes** to listening to what is right for your body.

Crunch Time on Healthy Snacks

Biscuits and crisps are irresistible as snacks because of their crunch factor, but they can be the downfall to any diet. Research[28] has been done to explain the compelling urge to wrap our gums around something crunchy. Physicists at the Leeds University used an ultrasonic pulse echo technique (think whales and dolphins) in the measurement of the crispness of biscuits. Apart from explaining the Great Butterscotch Snap Shortage of 1981*, the team came to some juicy conclusions.

Basically, crunchy food sends a powerful ultrasound wave through our system which makes the eating experience even better. Apparently the wave triggers a reaction in the brain that causes a sensation of pleasure.

So assuming there's no helping our innate attraction to crunchy foods, at least aim for healthy options – apples, carrots, the chick pea mix detailed in Tool 7: Yummy Scrummy Mummy Love.

Here are some *healthy* crunchy foods:

- Low-fat popcorn;
- Rice cakes and rice crackers;
- Almonds, walnuts, pistachios;
- Raw capsicum sticks (surprisingly sweet!); and
- Baked multi-grain pretzels with sesame and poppy seeds

* fictitious

Checklist: 21 Tools for a Healthy Body

Refer to this checklist during your 21-day makeover and tick off each tool as you incorporate it into your plan. You may choose to do one tool many times, but aim to try them all at least once. On some days you will probably find you have incorporated up to six of them. That's OK. Also rate each tool for its ease, its suitability to your aptitude, and how likely you are to incorporate it into your daily life. (1 = unlikely, 5 = bring it on!) This way, if you're having trouble choosing your top tools (unlikely, but it's better to be prepared) you can go with your highest rating tools to make part of your daily lifestyle.

○ **Hara Hachi Bu** (Eat until you are 80 percent full)

  Date(s) incorporated:

  Make it part of my daily lifestyle? 1   2   3   4   5

○ **Enter the Carb-Free Zone** (Eat the right carbs)

  Date(s) incorporated:

  Make it part of my daily lifestyle? 1   2   3   4   5

○ **Abstain After Six** (Finish eating by 6pm)

  Date(s) incorporated:

  Make it part of my daily lifestyle? 1   2   3   4   5

○ **Lubricate It** (Drink at least two litres of water)

  Date(s) incorporated:

  Make it part of my daily lifestyle? 1   2   3   4   5

○ **Twice As Nice** (Double the exercise, double the fun)

  Date(s) incorporated:

  Make it part of my daily lifestyle? 1   2   3   4   5

O **Halvies Heaven** (Halve unnecessary food)

Date(s) incorporated:

Make it part of my daily lifestyle? 1   2   3   4   5

O **Yummy Scrummy Mummy Love** (Find comfort food)

Date(s) incorporated:

Make it part of my daily lifestyle? 1   2   3   4   5

O **Lighten Up** (Eliminate guilt)

Date(s) incorporated:

Make it part of my daily lifestyle? 1   2   3   4   5

O **In Your Own Good Time** (Enjoy slow food)

Date(s) incorporated:

Make it part of my daily lifestyle? 1   2   3   4   5

O **Friends With Fat** (Add good fats to your diet)

Date(s) incorporated:

Make it part of my daily lifestyle? 1   2   3   4   5

O **Empty the Waist Basket** (Flush toxins)

Date(s) incorporated:

Make it part of my daily lifestyle? 1   2   3   4   5

O **Renounce Pain** (Make exercise fun)

Date(s) incorporated:

Make it part of my daily lifestyle? 1   2   3   4   5

O **Oooh La La, Brad Pitt is Coming!** (Stand tall)

Date(s) incorporated:

Make it part of my daily lifestyle? 1   2   3   4   5

○ **Burnout Buster** (Balance your meals)

Date(s) incorporated:

Make it part of my daily lifestyle? 1   2   3   4   5

○ **Upside Down and Inside Out** (Eat a big breaky)

Date(s) incorporated:

Make it part of my daily lifestyle? 1   2   3   4   5

○ **Spice-It-Up** (Trust your body's messages)

Date(s) incorporated:

Make it part of my daily lifestyle? 1   2   3   4   5

○ **To Digest, Divine** (Consider digestive enzymes)

Date(s) incorporated:

Make it part of my daily lifestyle? 1   2   3   4   5

○ **Burn Baby Burn** (Increase incidental exercise)

Date(s) incorporated:

Make it part of my daily lifestyle? 1   2   3   4   5

○ **On the Wagon** (Limit your alcohol intake)

Date(s) incorporated:

Make it part of my daily lifestyle? 1   2   3   4   5

○ **Daylight Savings** (Adjust your time zone)

Date(s) incorporated:

Make it part of my daily lifestyle? 1   2   3   4   5

○ **Yes, yes, yes, yes, yes, yes and yes** (Yes to well-being)

Date(s) incorporated:

Make it part of my daily lifestyle? 1   2   3   4   5

Mind Over Matter

I see perfection

in my reflection

Once upon a time, Shrek, Brad Pitt and Angelina Jolie were having lunch together. Each of them were concerned that, although they'd all been described as the strongest, sexiest and most gorgeous of all time, how could they be sure?

They all decided that the best way to find out was to ask the famous talking Mirror Mirror on the Wall to confirm for them whether Shrek was the strongest, Brad was the sexiest and Angelina was the most gorgeous. They agreed to meet again the next day to discuss their findings.

The next day Shrek said with a smile, "Well, it's true. The mirror told me that I am the strongest man in the world."

Brad Pitt perked up and said, "And it confirmed for me that I'm the sexiest man alive."

But, Angelina Jolie lifted her sad, gorgeous face and said..."Who the hell is Anita Revel?"

The Most Beautiful Woman in the World

Last year I ran a poll on my website to find out who my visitors think is the most beautiful woman in the world. More than 500 women voted, with choices ranging from Madonna, Lucy Liu to Sophia Loren and others. In a decisive victory, 62 percent of the women voted that the most beautiful woman in the world is… "in the mirror!"

It is very heartening that this result shows countless women are able to recognise their own beauty as valuable and valid. One reason for this may be that they challenge the implication that skinny/rich/celebrity is the only 'sexy'. As any girl who has read a gossip magazine knows, it can be intimidating to look at the Size Zero swanettes in their swanky clothes, glossy hair and flash cars – it can make a girl feel a little inadequate and frumpy compared with their apparently glamorous lives.

But when I looked a little closer at this subliminal message that women must be skinny, rich and shallow to be successful, this is what I found.

- In 2007, a young socialite freaked out about the prison-issue beauty products – a bar of soap. If she were in touch with her inner goddess, she'd know that eight glasses of water each day is generally enough to nourish her skin, organs, mind and attitude. Water fills out your wrinkles (aka 'laugh lines') and makes your skin glow with natural health.
- Certain fashionistas renowned for their size zero wardrobes, are reportedly losing their hair. If they were in touch with their inner goddess they'd know to eat a beautiful variety of fruit, vegetables, wholegrains, nuts, seeds and protein every day to nurture their bodies, keep them alert, strengthen their bones and nails and give their hair a healthy shine.

- Some actresses exercise so much they are in danger of having an obsession-related syndrome named after them. If they were in touch with their inner goddess they'd be happy with only 30 minutes of moderate exercise every day to keep their blood flowing, their metabolism firing, their immune system strong and their fitness at a level to keep them strong indefinitely.

- The paparazzi love focusing on boob jobs, botched facelifts, evidence of surgery and cosmetic boo-boos. If their subjects were in touch with their inner goddesses they'd understand that it takes more than big knockers, fake-up and plastic implants to be sexy. They'd understand every crease tells a story, every curve is defining, and that with age comes wisdom. They'd ditch what they *believe* is sexy, and reclaim their inner fabulous-and-free, luscious wild woman.

I have used this research in my modern-day story for well-rounded women, BOTIBOTO (*Beautiful On the Inside, Beautiful On the Outside*). It's for sale by donation from my website, but if you haven't read it yet, I can offer you this piece of advice in the meantime: **get real**!

I have real thoughts, real attitude
and real values. I am real,
I am heard, I matter and
I am reeeeaaaaal priceless!

Intentional Empowerment Tool: One Kind of Beautiful

Glamorous is beautiful, but beauty isn't just glamorous. Beauty is the new mother glow, the warmth between friends, the compassion in a helping hand, the curve of a hip, the aura of confidence. Flick through your favourite magazine and describe all the different kinds of beautiful.

Changing Your Mind

"What you say is what you are" is a catch-cry I've heard bandied about the schoolyard as a taunt. What a pity! Such negative messages absorbed in our formative years manifest as limiting beliefs later on. The negative feelings become self-doubt, self-judgement and self-criticism.

It's ironic that the meaning behind the words was never intended to make children feel scared to open their mouths. The catch-cry stems from the adage originally coined by Buddha: "We are what we think. And that which we are arises with our thoughts. With our thoughts, we make our world."

Consciously shift any negative perceptions of the childhood taunt, and transform it into a phrase with positive intentions. After all, what is wrong with being what you say you are? Try owning this answer: "Yes, I am what I say I am, and I am absolutely wonderful!"

Your mind is a powerful machine. When you're in the driver's seat it's up to you how much abundance, love and joy you have in your life. Learning to reprogram your mind to think positively is the only tried-and-true way of cancelling out all the random noise that prevents you from realising your full potential. So change your mind to change your mind. When you can think positively, you can steer your intentions in a direction that proves beneficial for your highest good. Just how much you can transform your life is totally up to your imagination – literally. Remember your promise to make it easy.

Avoid the trap of Toxic Thinking – also known as the art of self-sabotage. Following are some tips for recognising toxic thoughts and ways to deal with them.

Toxic Thinking

Pondering about life and soul matters can lead to self-improvement, but when that pondering turns into a noisy headache of nagging thoughts, it's time to tone it down.

Dr Susan Nolen-Hoeksema, author of *Women Who Think Too Much* (Piatkus 2003) describes toxic thoughts as 'overthinking', the process that leads to the 'toxic triangle' – depression, binge eating, and binge drinking.

"When you are caught in overthinking, you go over your negative thoughts and feelings, examining them, questioning them, kneading them like dough," she says.

Are Your Thoughts Toxic?

- Can you accept help from others?
- Do you often think, "why can't I get going?"
- Are you fiercely independent and proud of it?
- Do your criticisms outweigh your compliments?
- Is it easier to complain about something than fix it?
- Are you afraid to let others see your vulnerable side?
- Have you had a loss that you haven't properly grieved?
- Does an imperfection prevent you from success?
- Do you rehash situations and wish they'd gone better?
- Have you had a major life change that wasn't given enough time to adjust?

If you answered 'often' or 'always' to most, you may be worrying about things rather than working on them.

Types of Toxic Thinking

There are three primary types of Toxic Thinking that are most common for us to engage in.

1. **Rant-And-Rave** "Rant-and-Rave is the most familiar type and usually centres around some wrong we believe has been done to us," says Susan. "Rants-and-Raves take on an air of wounded self-righteousness and focus on designing a retribution that will severely sting our victimisers."

   Thoughts such as, "I can't believe they would do this to me," can lead to impulsive choices along the lines of spontaneously resigning from a job, reckless retribution that you might later regret, or rash decision-making that backfires.

2. **Runaway Train** Runaway Train thoughts are those that take on a life of their own. They begin innocently as we ponder a recent event but begin to spiral out of proportion as we entertain possible causes for our feelings about the events. A thought such as "I'm feeling a bit low," leads to, "because I have no friends, or maybe it's because I haven't lost any weight this month, or maybe it's because of all those things that happened in my past."

   "I call these Life-of-Their-Own thoughts – they cause us to see problems that don't really exist, or at least aren't as big as our thoughts make them out to be," says Susan. "They can also cause us to make bad decisions about these problems we feel we have. We confront others, we decide to quit our job or school or we cancel social outings, acting out of our bad moods and exaggerated concerns."

3. **Random Rumbles** When you can't zero in on only one thing to think about, or focus on one issue in the quagmire of your thoughts, it leads to a feeling of being shut down and isolated. Buddhist monks call this state a 'monkey mind', when thoughts race around and create mental churn.

"Like a frog on a hot stove, Jumbled-Up thoughts occur when we don't move in a straight line from one problem to another," says Susan. "All kinds of concerns, many of them unrelated, flood our minds all at the same time."

People who drink alcohol or take drugs in response to this type of overthinking may be trying to drown out background noise that has been with them since childhood. This leads to a feeling of being immobilised and unable to see a clear path forward.

How to Detox Your Thoughts

If you keep thinking negatively, you will keep yourself confused, discouraged, vengeful and depressed. It is important to declare your own mind a battle-free zone, and to develop a zero tolerance for chronic negativity.

For anyone stuck in a pattern of toxic thinking, it is possible to escape and reclaim your direction by turning negative thoughts into positives. There are three important steps in detoxifying such patterns and becoming the director of your own emotional life.

1. **Break the Grip**   The first step is to break the grip of the thoughts with short-term strategies such as taking a break with an active distraction – going for a walk, talking with a trusted counsellor, or socialising with friends.

   Leonie Young, CEO of beyondblue: the national depression initiative, says, "Meeting other women for fun and enjoyable activities not only boosts motivation, it provides a social environment for us to communicate, share ideas and problem-solve. Ultimately this leads to an increased sense of belonging, reduced isolation and assists us to deal with whatever life throws at us."

Susan Nolen-Hoeksema's research shows that as little as eight minutes is enough to break the cycle of repetitive thought. She also found that once that pattern was broken and the over-thinker was doing something pleasant, it made her mood more positive, enabling her to think clearer and actually solve the problem.

2. **Move to Higher Ground** "Stop waiting around to be rescued," says Susan. "Gain a new perspective and begin problem-solving, using strategies such as feel your pain and move on."

   One way to do this is by carving some time for yourself to observe toxic thoughts as they manifest. Learn to recognise what your thoughts are doing. Take time. Easy does it. Be gentle, and be prepared to address the root of the sabotaging thought rather than reacting to its toxicity.

   Do something small to start with, such as joining the 'thought police' and mentally yelling "STOP!" when you find toxic thoughts creeping in. Visualising a stop sign will help reinforce the signal to your subconscious to give it a rest.

3. **Avoid Future Traps** Aim for long-term changes in your life to avoid future bouts of self-sabotage. One way to begin is to develop multiple sources of self-esteem and emotional support. Listen for others' voices – the voices of family, friends, and pop culture that support you in a positive way to feel and act.

   Something to be wary of, however, is to avoid well-meaning friends who only emote with you – this could convince you even more that you're right to be so negative. And one last piece of advice from Susan: "Stop worrying so much!"

Bring On The ATTITUDE!

When I was child, a guardian complained that I had too much *Attitude*. With a capital A. So it's not surprising that for years I though Attitude was a bad thing. Then I woke up. Now, when I apply Attitude to achieve my highest good, Attitude is a *fabulous* thing! A positive attitude is life-saving. A can-do attitude gets things done. And a healthy attitude kicks ass tae-bo style. Yeeee-haaaaaaa.

Do you see how easy that was? I simply changed my mind about my attitude to Attitude! I rejected someone else's implication that Attitude is a bad thing and adopted my own healthy and pro-active Attitude that serves me to this day. My Attitude has morphed from something that annoyed my guardian, to an acronym representing essential values that I hold sacred today:

A	Affirmative Action
T	Tolerance
T	Truth
I	Individualism
T	Trust
U	Unconditional Love
D	Daily Salutes
E	Easy Does It.

If you haven't already started a journal, here is your first exercise. Although we'll be exploring my Attitude values in this section, I want to you concurrently explore your own values that *you* hold sacred. Perhaps they'll form an acronym of a word you'd like to reframe, too. Just as I found practical ways to instil each value in daily life, find ways to 'walk your talk' via intentional pursuits. There are over 300 values listed in *The Goddess DIET Companion* to get you started, or use your own journal, and begin!

Affirmative Action

By the time you go to bed tonight, you will have had around 60,000 thoughts go through your head. Reflect on your day for a moment… what ratio of your thoughts were positive? Were they mostly random or deliberate? Were they out of left-field or in reaction to a catalyst?

Just think how lovely it would be if you could answer that 100 percent of your conscious thoughts were positive? And even lovelier if your subconscious ones were too! I would also hope that a fair portion of your thoughts were devoted to a beautiful Affirmation and/or Creative Visualisation, but if this hasn't been the case so far, fear not – we are about to learn more about these valuable tools for mental health.

Affirmations

Affirmations are a very simple tool that prove very effective in changing and empowering your mindset for positive results. I have been using them for more than 15 years now with stunning results – they have helped me achieve happiness in many aspects of my life.

An affirmation is a short, positive statement that describes an ideal outcome of a wish. By identifying what you want from your life and expressing it in words as though it has already come to fruition, you are sending a clear message to the Universe of what you want to receive. A successful affirmation has three elements:

1. A clear sense of purpose: Your affirmation must be a dedicated belief, not an ad hoc approach to 'trying it out'. Apply your full commitment and purpose when you ask for what it is you wish to achieve.

2. Trust: Believe without fear or guilt that your desire is closer to fruition each time you say it. Trust that what

is right for you is on its way. Know that you truly
deserve what you are asking for and be ready to
accept it.

3. Perseverance: Repeat your affirmation dozens of
    times daily, seven days a week, until the belief
    becomes part of your DNA and your desire manifests
    as reality. *Never quit*. The rewards outweigh the effort.

There are many variations and outcomes possible. And
there are many ways to keep affirmations happening
every day. They can be spoken out aloud, recorded in
your private diary repetitively, or written on individual
sticky notes and hung around your daily environment. Be
creative in how you get your affirmations happening so
they're always top of mind.

How to Create Your Own Affirmation

Imagine that a genie has popped out of a bottle and
granted you a wish. Perhaps you asked to lose weight.
Instead of focusing on your bathroom scales, focus on
how you feel after the magic wand has been waved and the
wish fulfilled. Are you now comfortable in your body
and clothes? Are you feeling fitter? Stronger? More alive?

The secret to successful weight loss (and health gain) lies
within losing attachment to ugliness, self-criticism and
self-loathing. Rather than focussing on a dress size or
other specific details (that will only serve to disappoint
you if you are unable to reach the goal), anchor your
affirmation on your emotions and feelings upon
succeeding. You might say, "I feel sexy in my clothes that
are exactly right for me." This way, it doesn't matter what
size or weight you are, it only matters that you feel
fabulous in whatever state of curvaliciousness.

Your affirmation should always be written in present
tense. Using words like 'will do' keeps your outcome in

the future out of your reach. It must also be written using positive words – the Universe does not acknowledge words such as 'not'. For example, if you say "I am not poor" the Universe hears "I am poor". Ask instead for, "I have enough money for all that I need."

Positive thoughts attract positive energy.

Get Real About Your Affirmation

If you decide that you are tired of looking in the mirror and seeing a worn-out, frumpy old hag in it, you might decide to make your affirmation, "I am beautiful." This way you'll begin to notice your sparkling eyes, knock-em-out smile and the years of wisdom that lie beneath the layers of wrinkles. Right?

But what *really* happens when you look yourself in the eye and say, "I am beautiful"? What you hear in your head after you've said your affirmation is the *real* affirmation.

If this little voice is laughing, scoffing or challenging your statement, it is overriding your healthy intentions. It's working to trash your success. In short, because this negative message is the last thing you heard, this is the message you'll end up acting upon!

In other words, it's these back-enders that are really setting the tone for your success. If you're good at self-trashing, then you probably won't even hear the back-enders at first.

To hear them it's just a matter of listening for them. If you're an expert at self-trashing, your back-enders will be yelling at you at a deafening roar. In fact, they'll be turned up to '11' on the Spinal Tap scale. The self-talk might go something like this:

You: I am beautiful

Your back-ender: NO YOU'RE NOT! Who do you
                       think you are? Can't you see the
                       saggy skin? Try some orange peel
                       on those thighs. Where the hell did
                       all those wrinkles come from?

The idea is to retrain your back-enders to sing a positive
tune. Consciously instruct your self-talk to follow
protocol to agree with your affirmation. For example,

You: I am beautiful

Your back-ender: Yeah, I see it! My eyes are flecked
                       with magic, my dimples are deeper
                       than ever, and I am totally beauty-
                       FULL! Love the hair I've got goin'
                       on today. Good job! Yummy curves
                       happenin' today… way to go,
                       goddess! This colour really suits
                       me, I love how it highlights my
                       eyes. And pose! Oh yeah, check out
                       the power babe in the mirror.
                       Knock 'em dead you bootylicious
                       stunwana. Deliver me into
                       succulent joy, you radiant shining
                       star. (And so on…)

Persevere with training the little critic in your head to
work with you rather than against you.

If you choke on the glowing endearments to your
reflection, see this as a sign you have hit the sweet spot of
your critic. Yippee, you can now paint a big red target
around this issue and deal with it accordingly. When you
stop choking over your self-validations, congratulations,
you have harnessed your inner-critic's powers and can
now start using them for good.

Creative Visualisation

Creative Visualisation is a form of meditation that allows you to imagine yourself achieving your desires. Author Shakti Gawain[29] brought this concept to the forefront of consciousness over 25 years ago, but the practice has been around for centuries. Jesus, for example, referred to the power of creative thinking when he said, "Whatsoever things you desire when you pray, believe that you receive them and you shall have them."

The key word here is *believe*. Or as I prefer to say, *trust*. You can use Visualisation to release negative experiences in your past that have you believing you deserve hardship, obstacles and problems. Use this time to think again and believe/trust that you deserve an incredible, joyful and easy journey. Trust that you can surrender your fixation on a particular object or desire, and that the Universe will provide that which is exactly right for you.

Before Building Your Creative Visualisation

To get a positive outcome, keep your thoughts vibrating at a positive level. Instead of seeing 'ugly' in the mirror, change the tape and say beautiful things about yourself. Instead of feeling clumsy at dinner parties see yourself as the shining star. Quit beating up on yourself and claim your joy! Here are some more tips to achieve a successful Visualisation.

1. **Set Your Goal – Not**

   Goal-setting is a concept that gets bandied about so often I almost can't hear it anymore. I think one of my colleagues Maria Elita[30] is the only life coach in the world who doesn't agree with goal-setting – it's too easy to set your sights on something you *think* you need rather than what you *really* need. Through my own life experiences, I agree with her. Too often I achieved a goal that I had listed and striven for only to feel deflated once I achieved it. Like a dog who actually catches a car, the inevitable response to achieving a goal is, "What now?" What an anti-climax!

What car you drive doesn't matter; only feeling proud in how you get from Point A to B does. The size label on your clothes doesn't matter; feeling foxy in your clothes does. So instead of writing a list of *things* you'd like to achieve or things you'd like to *own*, simply describe how you'd like to *feel* when you've got it.

Make this *feeling* your goal rather than pre-conceived ideas about objects or situations that you expect will bring you happiness. Resist being greedy or materialistic – driving a status car or being a size zero is not the key to your happiness.

When visualising how you intend to feel, clarify that it is for your highest good, and that it is what you really need (rather than what you *think* you need).

2. Be committed

For change to happen, you must commit to it. Think of your last New Year's resolution for example. Did you reel off the same resolution to become a sax goddess, or did you pick up the phone and book your first saxophone lesson? (Does anyone have Brad Pitt's phone number? My resolution to have his babies is 10 years old now.)

One study[31] found that people who had committed to their new year's resolution were 10 times more likely to succeed than those who had simply wished for a change to happen. Ergo, you must *act* for it to happen.

In practical terms, you are possibly asking "what's the difference between a wish and a commitment?" The easy answer is that wishing is passive while commitment is active. There's that word again: *act*.

If you *wish* for good health, it *may* come your way (along with your fairy godmother and a bowl of apples). This type of thinking is literally 'wishful thinking'. If your wishful thinking doesn't come true then it's unlikely you really care either way – you'll just put the lack of success down to "oh well, it wasn't meant to be." This is your way of saying you're powerless to help yourself (yawn) but it's not your fault (yawn again).

If you are committed to good health, on the other hand, you'll put down that deep-fried chicken drumstick right now and walk to the fruit store yourself. You care about the outcome because you have invested effort and intention into it. You haven't waited for things to happen magically, and you haven't given it a half-hearted go with a flippant comment such as "Let's just see how this pans out." You've been proactive, acted with consciousness, and given yourself every chance to taste, feel, see, hear and enjoy success.

When going through your creative visualisation exercise, put yourself in the 'committed' mindset. You'll get nowhere by yawning at the end of your little visual journey and saying, "Oh wouldn't that be nice, but won't happen in my lifetime." (Ouch, there's that back-ender again.) I'd love a dollar for every time I heard, "Other people are lucky; I'm not." Turn your luck around. Put yourself right in the picture and bask in how good it feels to be doing something to fix a crappy situation. Which leads me to…

3. Put Yourself in the Picture

Mentally see, hear or feel yourself enjoying the
outcome of your goal. See yourself walking to the
fruit store every day. Taste how *good* the fresh produce
is. Feel how wonderful it is to have fresh air in your
lungs and a youthful glow to your cheeks...

Don't worry about *how* you're going to lose those
60 gadzillion kilograms of baggage. Just see your
clothing becoming easier and easier to wear. See
yourself playing with your kids on the beach for
longer and longer periods. Feel how much more
energy you have the more you move. Enjoy glorious
sex thanks to your new Attitude. Feel how easy it is to
smile because *finally* you are choosing joy over sorrow
and hardship.

Know that because you have asked for your highest
good, and that you're willing to act upon your
commitment, the Universe will provide.

Do this every hour (more: every minute, or less: every
day) until you program yourself to believe that what
you're seeing is not only your reality, but your
birthright. It won't take long before it *is* your reality
and you'll be wondering, "why the heck didn't I do
this earlier?!" You go girl!

The Right Way to Do a Creative Visualisation

Oh please, if there was a 'right way' to do anything we'd
all be doing it that way and there would be no diversity.
That would be like living a vanilla life. Yick!

The beauty about humanity is that we're all unique.
There is no such thing as one size fits all, so consider this
your permission to create the visualisation that suits you
perfectly.

Seeing as you're unique, your visualisation is just as unique. Tailor it to fit you exactly, and to serve you exactly. It doesn't need to be complex or detailed. It can be five minutes long, fifty minutes long, or just eight seconds if that is right for you. It can be written, recorded or drawn on story cards. In fact, each of us has a predominant method for learning so use whichever one of these methods that comes naturally.

1. **Auditory**: The auditory person hears their Creative Visualisation with words and sounds. It might sound like a first-person narrative running through your head, or that you're being told a story in third-person, or that you're being presented with a series of sounds or snippets of music that make up a montage visualisation.

2. **Visual**: Visual people can see vivid and detailed pictures or images in their mind. It might play like a movie in your head, or be a series of photos where you can see yourself achieving your goal.

3. **Kinaesthetic**: The kinaesthetic person can feel the emotions associated with achieving their goals. If you're kinaesthetic, you'll be able to feel what it is like to win, to fall in love, or the lightness that comes when pain released.

Some tips for success

- Hit Replay. Keep your visualisation at the forefront of your thoughts, and replay the visualisation many times every day. If you are busy, you can play snippets at a time. There's no need to be rigid in your starting point or sequence – you could simply skip to the bit you're stepping out with your shoulders back and feeling like a million dollars. Or at least to the bit where you have just earned your first million dollars.

- Trust. Override deep-seated negative programming, and think positively towards the scenario in your visualisation. Denial or doubt only serves to reinforce negative vibrations so train yourself to truly believe that you deserve what you are asking for. Feel what is happening as you internalise your success and realise the certainty of your Visualisation being fulfilled.

- Don't over-analyse. If you are presented with thoughts or feelings you don't understand, don't be distracted by trying to interpret meanings. Just relax and accept that the answer will reveal itself in due course.

- Release toxic thoughts. Sometimes you will find your mind reverting to old habits of self-sabotage. It may try and override your success with negative statements such as "this is ridiculous!" or "oh come on, who in their right mind would really love me?" Visualise a stop sign and show it to your inner critic. Let your mind know that you are releasing negativity and welcoming joy.

- As goals can change before they are realised, be gentle on yourself if you evolve into a more positive being that realises you can aim higher than your original intention!

Persevere with your creative visualisation. Even if you don't achieve your goal in one day, one week or one month, at the very least you are on the path to surmounting negative patterns.

I'll be giving you suggested affirmations and visualisations throughout Part 3 of this book, but you're welcome to create your own based on what is right for you. (See how I'm handing the responsibility for your success back to you? Be empowered!)

Tolerance

For those of you who have been criticising your dimpled thighs for centuries, start noticing your perfections instead. Then, while your attention is diverted away from your 'imperfections' you can train your mind to be more tolerant about aspects of yourself that you believe (rightly or wrongly) are ugly.

Why do you think your body parts are ugly anyway? Every guy I know *loves* curves in a woman, yet quite a few women who participate in a Goddess Playshop™ [32] express a wish to be thinner. Or to at least lose their jelly belly, spare tyre, love handles, cankles... the list of self-criticisms goes on. There are *many* reasons for this mindset in the first place, but you'll feel it change as soon as you challenge any message that there is a 'right' body shape. The only 'beautiful' body shape is that which is right for you. Never compare yourself with a model who has been professionally made up, airbrushed, digitally enhanced and who has possibly skipped a meal or two – this is only one type of 'beautiful'. You are another type of 'beautiful' as is your sister, boss, aunty and niece. Celebrate the million types of 'beautiful'.

Give up any fixation with the highly stylised version of 'beauty' that we see in music videos, in fashion spreads and on the red carpet. I offer you these words of wisdom from TV host Judge Judy. In a classic statement that implies that personality always trumps appearances, she declared, "Beauty fades. Dumb is forever."

Remember we are all unique – and how lucky that we are. Can you imagine being a clone of your neighbour and living in the same solar-insensitive, eco-guzzling house? Or going clubbing and wearing the same dress as your friends because that's *the* dress made to suit *the* standard body shape? Diversity is cool.

In an online poll I asked visitors how they feel when they read gossip magazines. Visitors could choose from: a) wish I were size zero, b) wish I were richer, c) want to be younger, d) realise I'm lucky and d) am grateful I'm perfect.

Over 60 percent of respondents said they realised they were lucky and were grateful they're perfect, while only 14 percent wished they could be a size zero. It seems women would rather be skinny than richer (10 percent), and a mere four percent wished they were younger. Good to see that 96 percent of visitors value the wisdom and rich experiences gained while growing (b)older.

Here are some examples for transforming a perceived imperfection into a positive attitude about your body. Make it an Intentional Empowerment Tool by listing your own 'uglies' in your journal and ways you can see them differently.

Perceived Ugliness	Becomes...
My butt is big	I have plenty of 'woman' for my lover to grab on to
My thighs are dimply	My hips are the perfect shape for my designer skirt
I have piano-leg ankles...	...that look great in knee-high boots
My belly is too round	All the better for belly-dancing with
I'm a size too big	Bring on the Botticelli revolution
I have an ugly nose	And it suits my gorgeous face just perfectly

Intentional Empowerment Tool: Serenity Prayer

This version of the Serenity Prayer is designed to improve your tolerance levels. When you realise that there are some things simply beyond your control, it's a lot easier to accept them and move on.

Which old habit do I want to release?

What is one thing that I **do** want to change?

Which new habit do I want to adopt?

What are things that I **don't** want to change?

What is my first step in order to achieve this?

Spirit please grant me the power of water to accept the things I cannot change, the power of fire to change the things I can, the power of air to know the difference of what I can and can't change, and the power of earth to handle the situation with love.

What are some things I **cannot** change?

When will I start?

If it takes 21 days to change a habit, what is my timeline?

Start here

When I am successful, what does my life look like?

Truth

A truthful woman is one who doesn't lie about anything except her age, weight, and her husband's salary. Nor does she blame her dry-cleaner for her pants being too tight, but we'll leave that to her discretion. In fact, a poll for the health magazine Prevention[33], found that 85 percent of American women would rather reveal their age than their weight – and even then they were likely to shave an average of four years off their age.

This is something I've never understood. Why tell someone you're 40 when you're really 44? So that they can think "gee, she has *not* aged well!" Why not tell them you're 50 and impress their socks off at how young you look? Or, why not just be proud of the truth? Ha! Now there's a novel idea!

Seriously now, sometimes we make up our own truths to help us deal with situations, and often we do this subconsciously. The problem with such self-talk is that it often feels like it is our truth. When the truth is distorted, it becomes dangerous.

You can't always control the situation you're in – a friend won't return your phone calls, for example – but you *can* control the way you react to it. You can halt any self-talk from turning negative ("Oh poop, she is angry with me, I am such a bad person.") and accept that the truth will reveal itself in time. (She got held up in meetings.)

Until the truth does present itself, your job is to accept that any negative self-talk is merely perception, not fact.

The Foundation For Life Sciences has a great fact sheet[34] for taking control of your thought processes, which is also accessible from Reach Out[35] (an initiative of the Inspire Foundation).

I'm about to spill some goss here. It concerns a good friend of mine. Gather around girls! (What is it about gossip that has us pricking up our ears and listening intently? Sigh... more on that in a moment.)

My friend, whom I shall call Tizzy for the sake of this story, used to have a bad habit of hearing something in conversation then repeating is as fact a few days later.

"Where did that information come from Tiz?" I'd ask. "Is this fact or is it a Chinese whisper?"

That would always stump her. Only when I asked her to clarify the legitimacy of her 'facts' did she think to question them or their source. Before that, she was happy to take idle talk on board and make the contents of that hearsay her reality. Not only could this be damaging for any people the information pertained to, it was lazy not to check any further for the truth.

Which brings me back to the very human habit of gossip. Mindlessly repeating hearsay as truth can be tactless, unnecessary and sometimes pretty nasty. In all my years of working with goddess archetypes, I have yet to find a tattletale amongst them. Therefore I can safely say mindless prattle is definitely not goddess-like behaviour.

So, before you spread 'truth' about yourself or someone else, well intended or otherwise, ensure that the words leaving your mouth are your truth. Too often we say what we think others want to hear – usually to keep the peace or to avoid rocking the boat. Enough of that. Step up to own your truth, goddess sister, and be proud of every word you say. Honour your goddess within by expressing your needs and desires with tact and honesty. Know that each time you tell your truth and act in accordance with your truth, you are using a very effective Intentional Empowerment Tool for your well-being.

Intentional Empowerment Tool: Revise Your Truth

This is a useful and easy exercise that I do when I need help with putting a truth into words. Simply identify a self-limiting belief (such as, "I am hopeless") and create a new constructive belief for yourself ("I am worthy").

Brain: Negative thought about a
situation creates a limiting belief

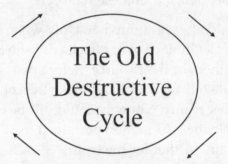

Outcome:
Hardship is
manifested
in response
to auric
signal. Life
is hard.

Body:
Negative
vibration
through
meridian,
organs and
chakras

Aura: Reflects dis-ease in body,
radiates negativity to the Universe

Brain: Positive thought about a
situation creates unlimited potential

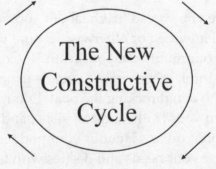

Outcome:
Joy and
success is
manifested
in response
to auric
signal. Life
is easy.

Body:
Positive
vibration
through
meridian,
organs and
chakras

Aura: Reflects balance in the body,
radiates abundance to the Universe

Old belief _____

_____

What this
belief
manifests
for me

_____
_____
_____

**The Old
Destructive
Cycle**

How this
belief makes
me feel

_____
_____
_____

How I appear to others

_____
_____

New belief _____

_____

What this
belief
manifests
for me

_____
_____
_____

**The New
Constructive
Cycle**

How this
belief makes
me feel

_____
_____
_____

How I appear to others

_____
_____

Individualism

Here are some inspiring words about being an individual from an interesting source: Dr Seuss.

> *"Be who you are and say what you feel, because those who mind don't matter and those who matter don't mind."*

If we were designed to be the same as one another, we'd all have the same size nose, the same hair lustre and the same penchant for Thai food. Biochemically speaking, you are different from every other person who ever was or ever will be. You are also as unique as your fingerprints in your personality, appearance, and even in the way you process your food or appreciate k.d. lang music.

So being individual isn't something worth fighting against. What is worth fighting *for*, on the other hand, is the freedom and confidence to assert your individuality with style and grace.

"Cherish forever what makes you unique, 'cuz you're really a yawn if it goes!" says Bette Midler, and she's absolutely right. What makes you unique is what makes you (and everyone around you) sing. And now I'm speaking on behalf of the collective 'we' as I say, we want to take notice of what you'll do next, what gifts you'll bring to our lives, and how we'll be grateful that you chose to give us a peek of your authentic self.

Being proud of your unique character, views on life and natural-born talents increases your sense of significance, and how much perceived value you place on your self-worth. You're more likely to feel like you're contributing to your environment because in honouring your true You, you are offering your true You to others. And bringing joy to others feels rewarding.

Someone who feels unworthy of this does the opposite –
they wait for instructions on how to behave, what choices
to make and feel more comfortable by swimming with
the stream. Only dead fish swim with the stream,
goddess sister, so wake up, take a breath, and begin to
capitalise on all the things that make you different.

Enjoy these some tips on upholding your individuality
with flair.

- Be aware of your environment and spot ways in
  which you can add lustre and shine. For example:
  - You have to click your car's remote control to find
    your vanilla-brand car? Trade in your one-size-
    fits-all-mothers tank and get the car that sings
    your personality.
  - A neighbour's wild oats have taken over her front
    yard. Don your safety gear, fire up a whipper
    snipper and tame those wild oats! (Don't forget to
    yell yeeee-haaaaa – everything's so much more
    fun when you do).
  - You studied economics because your parents told
    you that being an artist is no way to make a
    living? Ah phooey, you know what to do… Your
    soul demands it, so you supply it!
- Break the rules occasionally. Wear red with green, find
  treasures at thrift stores, make comfy underwear the
  choix sexy du jour, and dye your hair whatever the
  heck colour you want it.
- Wave at the dead fish that are swimming *down*stream
  as you swim *up*stream. Peer pressure can be
  challenging in terms of fashion, career ambitions,
  mothering and social networks. Remember, **it is easy**
  to honour your intuition and make fashion, career,
  parenting and friend choices that are exactly right for
  you. If the shoe fits… *strut it!*

- Watch out for the three baddies of individuality: arrogance, jealousy and the 'optometrist disease' – a fixation with I, I, I. (Sorry, bad pun on eye, eye, eye.)

  - Strive for a mixture of confidence and humility. Look for opportunities to learn about your world, while being proud of what you have learned already.

  - Use jealous remarks ("who does she think she is?") as opportunities to validate the achievements and good qualities of the person in question.

  - Avoid the spotlight occasionally – talking about yourself obsessively in conversations is *boring*. Listen for clues in your companion's conversation to use as fodder for questions and deeper interaction.

- Focus on your strengths – make your 'good' better, and your 'better' best. If you are unaware of what your strengths could be, ask your support circle – "What do you love most about me?" If you don't like what they say, no worries – it's not personal. Use the advice constructively and aim to improve in these areas if the advice rings true for you.

- "Well-behaved women rarely make history," says historian Laurel Thatcher Ulrich. It feels delicious stepping outside of a perception of how 'good girls' should behave – what are you going to do to be remembered for? (*Pssst!* Keep it safe!)

"Always be a first rate version of yourself instead of a second rate version of somebody else."

~ Judy Garland

Intentional Empowerment Tool: I am...

Write your name in the middle of this page – be big and bold! Be creative as you write down all the wonderful and positive adjectives you can think of that start with the first letter of your name... splash them all over the page in coloured texta, or cut the words out of magazines and create a collage. From these words, create an amazing affirmation starting with "I am..." that describes the gorgeous individual that you are.

Write your new Personal Power Statement below:

_____

_____

Trust

Mindlessly repeating, absorbing or believing 'facts' without question isn't always in your best interests. A modern goddess always consults her intuition – her ultimate source of wisdom – to work out what's right for her. Here's an example of how my intuition screamed "what?!" when I was presented with a supposed truth from a reputable source recently.

This particular source is an online initiative that exists to boost self-esteem and opportunities for youth. It may be a fabulous cause with noble intentions, but I was very surprised one day to surf onto their website and read on their home-page, "Only about five to 10 percent of women are in the height and weight range of models."

Alarm bells rang for me straight away. This 'fact' was credited to an Australian author whose work I love and believe to be credible, yet I found this statement very hard to swallow. For one thing, I have hundreds of friends in my network and *maybe* one or two would be in the height and weight range of a model. If the statistic were true, five to 10 percent of my 200 friends (that is, 10 – 20 women) could be strutting a catwalk for a living.

Five to 10 percent of women are in the height and weight range of models? What a dangerous and unsubstantiated statistic – it is basically saying that one in 10 to 20 girls should be tall and slim. Or, in a classroom of 30 girls, three are model material. REALLY?

When you 'see' a little red flag over an issue, or you 'hear' alarm bells about a situation, this is your intuition giving you the heads-up that the truth being presented to you may be incorrect. This is where **Trust** comes into play… Trust your intuition, your inner knowing, at all times.

Buddha has an excellent teaching about trust:

> *Believe nothing just because a so-called wise person said it.*
> *Believe nothing just because a belief is generally held.*
> *Believe nothing just because it is said in ancient books.*
> *Believe nothing just because it is said to be of divine origin.*
> *Believe nothing just because someone else believes it.*
> *Believe only what you yourself test and judge to be true.*
>
> – Buddha

More often than not, women in my generation were educated in left-brain dominated curricula – maths, science, and in my case, even religious instruction was taught by formula. Art, drama and other right-brained pursuits were generally considered electives, or not as essential in real life skills. But what this style of education did was teach us to think logically rather than foster creativity. We learned to live in our heads and we lost touch with our bodies, our signals, and our receptors to the greater environment. We became disconnected with our authentic and powerful selves – our primal connection to Mother Earth and her nurturing gifts. Learning to trust your own wisdom begins with re-connecting to your authentic power. This power is your birthright, your god/dess-given gift, and your most effective guide for your beautiful journey.

The first step in *trusting* your intuition is learning how to *hear* or *feel* your intuition. For some people it is a voice, for others a sense, and for others a physical reaction. Sometimes it's all three at once. If you are new to listening out for your intuition, here is one very simple way to hear or sense it. I recommend this technique to intuitive newcomers, (ha ha, as if you're new to it!) It is an approach I used when deciding whether to move to Western Australia, which turned out to be a wonderful move, so I can guarantee its effectiveness. The technique?

Tossing a coin. Yep, tuning in to your intuition can be that easy. Here is how to do it:

1. Ask yourself a question that can only have a 'yes' or a 'no' answer;
2. Assign 'yes' to heads, 'no' to tails;
3. Toss the coin and consciously register, heads or tails?

When you see your answer represented by either heads or tails, feel what your body is doing. Is your gut churning? Is your heart jumping with excitement? Is a voice wailing "noooo!" or is it singing "yes!"? Or perhaps you are itching to toss it again until you get a different answer?

If you're feeling disappointed then you know the true answer to your question – the opposite to how the coin landed. But if your head is singing "yes!" then you also know the true answer to your question – it is according to how the coin did land.

Now listen... the coin didn't give you your answer. *You* did. You simply used the coin as a tool for understanding your intuition, and from your intuition you got your direction. Intuition is a powerful kind of inner wisdom. It's not necessarily rational or logical, and it's often no more than a hunch or an instinct. Sadly, many of us were raised to shut down these messages with a flippant, "Oh, I'm being silly," or we override the flashes with a derogatory "People will think I'm crazy." It's *so* important that you reclaim your connection with your most reliable source of judgement and insight. In continuing to deny your ingrained wisdom you are only serving to perpetuate feelings of unworthiness and insecurity.

For this reason, try this exercise to get reconnected...

Write down your immediate response to the following
questions. Don't dilly-dally or allow your left-brain to
interfere with logic or criticisms.

Cheesecake or chocolate brownie?

_____

At this moment, what do you fear the most?

_____

What is stopping you from living your dream?

_____

What is the most satisfying thing you've ever done?

_____

What do you need the most in all the world?

_____

Your answers hold valuable clues in where to start
making positive changes in your life. (Sorry, but the
cheesecake or brownie question was just a red herring to
get you flowing.)

In The Goddess DIET, tune into what your body is telling
you when it comes to your food choices. Your body is a
marvellous machine that monitors the amount of
nutrients it has and sends you messages when it needs
more energy (hunger) or certain types of food (cravings).
It even sends you messages when certain types of food
don't agree with it (allergic reactions).

So trust your intuition when it comes to what you
'should' be putting into your mouth.

Unconditional Love

Google the word love, and you get about 2.53 billion
results in 0.05 seconds. Then there are the sub-categories:
love poems, love quotes, meaning of love, love letters,
love songs, love making and more. Just goes to show,
love is as bottomless and as endless as the widest ocean…
if love is an ocean, let me fall in!

Love is the Universe's greatest power, but like everything
in the Universe, it has a sacred balancing force: Fear.
I dare to borrow a quote from Isaac Newton to illustrate
this concept: for every action there must be an equal and
opposite reaction. Every choice, every thought, every
action or reaction, comes from one of two places in your
heart – love or fear. Be love, be loved. Be fear, be feared.

You know you are operating from a place of fear when
you have trust issues, you're unable to forgive something
or someone, you might be entertaining thoughts of
retribution, you are bearing guilt, you're suffering regret
or loss, or you're unable to feel empathy or compassion
for others. Outwardly, it might be that it's difficult to
make friends or feel comfortable or fulfilled in a romantic
relationship. In all these cases I've just described, all is
love in fear and war. Pull on your steel-cap boots goddess
sister 'coz it's time to kick fear to kingdom come.

Love love love. I love love. I love loving love. I love that
love is a happy place to be. I love that I can choose to be
in a place of love no matter how dire the news on TV, or
how scary the economic crisis, or how prevalent natural
disasters appear to be. I love that my heart chakra has a
G-spot that activates when I repeat: Grace, Generosity
and Gratitude. I love that I'm surrounded by blessings
because I choose to count them. And I love that the more
I love love, the more unconditional it becomes.

In my experience, all that most women really want in a relationship, be it with a man, woman or platonic friendship, is pretty well the same thing: trust, respect, fun, passion, emotional availability, and above all, *ease*. Fair enough, they're all wonderful qualities to desire in a relationship. I suggest, however, that the key to success is that you see your *Self* as the most important person worthy of having a relationship with first. True friends, let alone Mr Right, aren't going to appear in your life if you're sending signals of self-loathing, insecurity, and low self-worth. You will only attract true love when you have learned how to live it within yourself.

The secret to finding the deep, euphoric, all-accepting, all-out, unconditional and true love you are seeking, is within *you*. You must fall in self-love (or at least self-like) so that you may attract an equally loving, respectful and gorgeous circle of friends. Your own beautiful brand of love must first be emitted naturally and gracefully from you in order to attract it in equal measure. Therefore, you can only rely on yourself first and foremost in order to find true, rip-roaring unconditional love.

How much you are prepared to love yourself is a measure of how much someone else can love you. Self-acceptance, forgiveness, and appreciation is paramount. And you know you are ready to put yourself 'out there' when you are prepared to marry yourself.

Yes, if you think you're good enough to marry in a metaphorical sense, then you've reached the point where you can value and love yourself in all your aspects. You are equally accepting of both your light and shadow sides, your public and private faces, your secret desires and your celebrated talents. These are worth sharing and honouring in a self-wedding that is a beautiful way to declare your self-love.

Intentional Empowerment Tool: Marry Yourself

Here is a poetic step-by-step plan for making a long-term commitment to your self-worth and appreciation (aka marrying yourself.[36])

1.   Set Your Intention.

Work out what you want to achieve by listing the desirable qualities you want from a marriage. For example, "a lifelong commitment from a partner in a relationship that exudes happiness at every turn." Before you can expect this commitment from someone else, you must first promise that you will do everything in your power to give this to yourself, every day.

2.   Throw Out Self-Loathing

Looking in the mirror and criticising your imperfections? Laughing off compliments and dismissing nods to your brilliance? Flying under the radar so your super-stardom goes unnoticed? These are classic signs that you have a degree of self-loathing. Self-loathing only serves to block you from finding happiness within. When you radiate unhappiness, you attract unhappy people. Unhappy people are generally commitment-phobes. So learn to like yourself girlfriend, and repeat after me: "Self-loathing is for suckers."

3.   See Yourself As Goddess

Begin to notice your perfections when you look in the mirror. Receive compliments as graciously and copiously as you give them. Say "yes, yes, YES" a lot, with revellious and delightful energy. Practice shameless acts of joy and master joyous acts of shame. Affirm yourself daily with delicious words including magical, mystical, sparkling, juicy, ethereal, beautiful, intuitive, succulent, wild and divine. When you see yourself as Goddess, this is the gorgeous energy you radiate and hence, you begin to attract similarly gorgeous people into your life.

4. Be Your Own Best Friend

Tell yourself jokes. Spoil yourself rotten. Keep yourself entertained by doing what *you* want to do. Write down a promise to self that you will "never put baby in the corner." (Thanks Patrick Swayze for that one.) Flick friends that dare to support habits of self-loathing. Become a magnet to new friends that are a reflection of your perfection.

5. Create Your Day.

Now that you are your own little solar system and the brightest little star at the centre of your own cosmos, it is time to invite family and friends who love you as much as you love yourself, and to help you celebrate your rocking divinity. Picture your perfect ceremony in your head, see the smiling faces of your friends as they witness your joy, play with wedding vows until you have the perfect expression of your perfect self.

6. Let the Party Begin.

Set the date, find your venue, send out invitations, and let the celebration of your commitment begin. A perfect scenario is a girls' night in sharing stories, promising support, co-creating mementoes and eating yummy food. Or the opposite scenario, you might decide to have a girls' night out and shake your booty 'til dawn. Ramp this idea up a notch on the spiritual scale by dancing the sun to bed and drumming it up again. Yet another scenario might be a wedding-style walk down an aisle with a solemn vow being declared before a celebrant. Ultimately, it's *your* day, you can do whatever you want to. Sing, "It's my party, I'll... (rejoice)... if I want to!"

Getting Real About Loving Your Body

We talked earlier about the media, fashion houses and society at large perpetuating the myth that a beautiful woman is thin, young and rich. Well, Dove commissioned a study in 2005 and found that out of 3300 girls and women between the ages of 15 and 64 in 10 countries, 68 percent agreed that media and advertising set an unrealistic standard of beauty that they could not hope to achieve[37]. It's important to remember that yes, models are beautiful, but again, they are only one kind of beautiful.

Thankfully the air-brush was unheard of when Rubens, Botticelli and Bouguereau were creating their fabulous works. They have inspired countless modern day works such as *Venice Reconstituted* at Venice Beach (by California artist Rip Cronk, 1989, pictured right), or Baron Von Lind's stunning pin-ups, or the alluring burlesque performers that captivate audiences world-wide.

The rubenesque curves and ethereal goddess magnetism is a standard of beauty that you are absolutely capable of achieving. In fact, if you look hard enough in the mirror, I'm sure you'll find elements of the divine in there. If not, here are some tips on how to see a goddess in the mirror.

Activities: Beauty Is As Beauty Does

○ Begin by looking into a mirror several times every day. Hold your own gaze for a short period of time, and say meaningfully, "You are beautiful," or, "Hello beautiful goddess."

○ When you step out of the shower, create your own Personal Power Pose in the mirror. Start with your hands together over your head, relax your shoulders, and then move your arms, legs and body until you settle into a natural pose. Say directly to your gaze, "You are goddess."

○ This one might get you giggling, but that's OK. Start by framing your foot with your hands. Move your hands around it, saying "I love my foot, my beautiful foot." Repeat this for your calves, your knees, and for every part of your body until you get to the top, then notice how amazing you look.

○ Where your attention goes, energy flows. Focussing on a spare tyre only adds weight to the issue. Express gratitude to your beautiful bits by affirming your reflection, and watch these 'bits' take precedence. When you lose attachment to 'ugliness', it loses it grip on you. Your body can then settle into its own perfect size, naturally and beautifully.

Daily Salutes

One method I use to foster self-love and gratitude is by practising daily prayers and rituals, which I call Daily Salutes, to thank Spirit and the Universe for all my blessings (which I often call *blissings*).

One element of these Salutes is making a conscious promise to my Self that I am honouring and adoring my im/perfections and choices. This may involve a little ritual of repeating this Chakra Creed to my reflection in the mirror – usually as I'm brushing my teeth or moisturising. Mind you, if I've woken up feeling I need more, I put down my toothbrush and dedicate my full attention to Self by first looking deeply into my reflection. I address myself, "Good morning, goddess," then repeat this creed. I channelled this creed during a particularly draining book tour to restore my sense of purpose and my sense of Self, and offer it to you now.

> *I connect now to my great earth mother,*
> *to friends, family and support for each other;*
>
> *I offer love to my divine self,*
> *I am creative, abundant and full of health;*
>
> *Power up, oh magnificent me,*
> *I am brave, honest and love to be free;*
>
> *Love and joy to my compassionate self,*
> *As I give I receive endless love and help;*
>
> *My truth flows through my words,*
> *I speak with diplomacy, courage and I am heard;*
>
> *I recognise and trust my gift of insight,*
> *It tells me true and leads me right;*
>
> *Here's to love, joy and oneness with all,*
> *My connection with Spirit is all powerful.*

Here's another idea you can use for a Daily Salute... it's a ritual for health and self love, and a prayer for beauty.

Ritual For Health and Self Appreciation

You will need three candles – one each to represent your faith, your Self and your intention. You'll also need some carving tools (lino-cutting tools would be adequate, or the tip of some scissors), and your favourite essential oils – I suggest the Goddess-ence sacral chakra blend but please, use the blend that resonates with you on an intuitive level.

Carve the first candle with a symbol that represents your major source of inspiration – for example, it could be an Ankh, spiral, labyrinth, triple moon, pentacle, triskele, Brighid's cross or a Celtic knot (to name a few symbols) to represent your patroness goddess. It could be the Choku Rei symbol (from Reiki) to represent Spirit, the cross to represent Jesus, the OM symbol, the star and crescent, the Jain hand, the kokopelli, your totem animal or the name of your god/dess.

Carve your name and a symbol that represents You on the second candle (such as your zodiac sign or your birth date), and on the third candle, carve the symbol of Venus, the goddess of beauty and love.

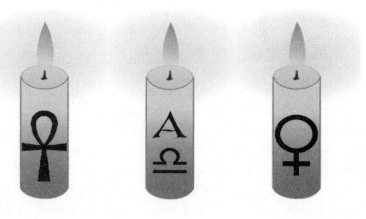

Each morning, anoint the first candle with your essential oils as you repeat the Prayer For Beauty (below). Light the candle as you complete the prayer to seal your intent, with particular emphasis on the first part of the prayer – this is the *asking* component of a successful affirmation. The next two parts of the prayer focus on the *believe* and the *receive* aspects of creating an affirmation, which we looked at earlier in Affirmative Action.

Repeat the process for the other two candles, only putting particular emphasis on the second part of the prayer when lighting the second candle, and the third part of the prayer for the third candle. When all three are alight and you are absolutely committed to achieving your success, offer your intentions to the Universe with the words, "I am ready to receive these blessings today." Blow the candles out to bring the ritual to a close.

Prayer For Beauty

I goddess, ask for the willpower to take charge of my life, my body and my habits, for the sake of my health, peace of mind and self-respect.

I goddess, believe my body is sacred, a treasure and pleasure, a luscious wonder and miraculous manifestation of the respect I have for my magnificent Self.

I goddess, am ready to receive blessings of dignity and grace during my transition, good health, and renewed energy to do anything I set my mind to.

Alternatively, make up your own prayer. Perhaps you could borrow inspiration from SARK's prayer pie from her *Juicy Living Cards* (Hay House 2003), that begins with "May you unfold willingly," and ends with "May you reach others with your radiant heart." Fill the middle of these two wishes with your own wonderful, wild wishes.

Easy Does It

To err may be human, but to purr is divine. And don't I just love purring?! I've got a purple suede lounge suite at the farm that I have set up to face the picture-glass windows overlooking the paddocks, rolling hills and adjacent forest. The sun spills in during the winter and forms a puddle over my lounge where it becomes a magnet to drenching myself in Goddess Time.

We all need a sacred space in our homes where we can *be*. A place to simply breathe, brood and let life go on around us. As well as a physical space to do this in, we need to give ourselves the permission and Goddess Time to enjoy our own company, our own insights and our own gifts.

Taking time to daydream, ruminate, percolate and germinate is as healthy for your body as a 30-minute physical workout. It clears cobwebs, refreshes perspective, recharges self-love and appreciation, helps you own the moment, and re-centres your view of yourself in the world. It is a form of meditation. Yes, even if you have a busy head, it's meditation. If you have read my book, *Sacred Vigilance*, you will have got the picture that I'm not a big fan of rule-ridden meditation. I believe you can connect easily with your unlimited potential within by unleashing your imagination and being as colourful or crazy or quiet as you want to be.

Being easy on yourself also entails releasing self-imposed expectations. Banish the word 'should' from your vernacular as this misleads you into thinking you need to be some-where other than your sacred space. If you catch yourself saying 'should', be honest: it's most probably something you don't really want to do at all. Free yourself from this burden and replace 'should' with 'could'. Hoooo, feels lighter already!

Intentional Empowerment Tool: Make a Love Mirror

When I ask friends how they spend their Goddess Time to rekindle their spark, answers range from "Read a book," to "Shoe shopping," to "Mountain-bike riding," to… and the list goes on. No matter what your relaxation style, next time you decide on Goddess Time, take an hour or so to immerse yourself in a bit of tinsel and glue to create yourself a Love Mirror. This will be your own personal mirror for you to use during The Goddess DIET when doing your affirmation and self-validation exercises.

What you will need:

- A mirror – it can be a compact, a wall mirror or in a free-standing frame for your bureau;

- A list of all the things you love about yourself;

- Glue, glitter, paints, feathers, sparkles, textas, carving tools, baubles, scissors and chocolate.

What to do:

- Decorate the mirror however you want to! Each time you apply a decoration onto the mirror's frame, say aloud something that you love about yourself. The mirror becomes the 'custodian' of all your finer points and will act as a tool for reminding you of how *good* you are no matter how *bad* things may be.

- Step two: Eat the chocolate.

Tips:

Consciously repeat your favourite affirmation, creed, motivating slogan, mantra or validation as you work. This will instil your mirror with a 'trigger' to remind you of this intention each time you pick it up.

Checklist: 21 Tools for a Healthy Mindset

You have just read many ideas and suggestions to realign your attitude from 'frump' to 'goddess' in the mirror. These are all Intentional Empowerment Tools for your mind and attitude. I have listed them here to remind you to use them ;-) You will find some of the tools only need doing once (such as the Make a Love Mirror tool), while others you can use every day.

○ **Read BOTIBOTO, Beautiful On The Inside Beautiful On The Outside, an Empowerment Story for Well-Rounded Woman** (Available by donation from botiboto.com)

   Date(s) incorporated:

   Make it part of my daily lifestyle?   1   2   3   4   5

○ **It Is Easy** (Consciously say this instead of "It's hard")

   Date(s) incorporated:

   Make it part of my daily lifestyle?   1   2   3   4   5

○ **See More Than One Kind of 'Beautiful'**

   Date(s) incorporated:

   Make it part of my daily lifestyle?   1   2   3   4   5

○ **Change Your Mind** (List of changes and strategies)

   Date(s) incorporated:

   Make it part of my daily lifestyle?   1   2   3   4   5

○ **Create Your Personal Values Acronym / Statement**

   Date(s) incorporated:

   Make it part of my daily lifestyle?   1   2   3   4   5

O **Master an Affirmation**

Date(s) incorporated:

Make it part of my daily lifestyle? 1 2 3 4 5

O **Create a Visualisation**

Date(s) incorporated:

Make it part of my daily lifestyle? 1 2 3 4 5

O **Demonstrate Tolerance** (Perceived 'ugly' becomes…)

Date(s) incorporated:

Make it part of my daily lifestyle? 1 2 3 4 5

O **Serenity Prayer**

Date(s) incorporated:

Make it part of my daily lifestyle? 1 2 3 4 5

O **Revise Your Truth** (Old versus New thought cycles)

Date(s) incorporated:

Make it part of my daily lifestyle? 1 2 3 4 5

O **Create an "I am…" Personal Power Statement**

Date(s) incorporated:

Make it part of my daily lifestyle? 1 2 3 4 5

O **Trust In Intuition** (Cultivate intuition)

Date(s) incorporated:

Make it part of my daily lifestyle? 1 2 3 4 5

O **Fall in Self-Love (**Commitment ceremony to Self)

Date(s) incorporated:

Make it part of my daily lifestyle? 1 2 3 4 5

O **"You Are Beautiful" Mirror Gazing**

Date(s) incorporated:

Make it part of my daily lifestyle? 1   2   3   4   5

O **Personal Power Pose**

Date(s) incorporated:

Make it part of my daily lifestyle? 1   2   3   4   5

O **Frame and Validate Parts of the Body**

Date(s) incorporated:

Make it part of my daily lifestyle? 1   2   3   4   5

O **Acknowledge Beautiful Bits**

Date(s) incorporated:

Make it part of my daily lifestyle? 1   2   3   4   5

O **Create Your Own Daily Salutes**

Date(s) incorporated:

Make it part of my daily lifestyle? 1   2   3   4   5

O **A Personal Ritual for Healing and Self-Appreciation**

Date(s) incorporated:

Make it part of my daily lifestyle? 1   2   3   4   5

O **Easy Time** (Find Goddess Time every day)

Date(s) incorporated:

Make it part of my daily lifestyle? 1   2   3   4   5

O **Make a Love Mirror**

Date(s) incorporated:

Make it part of my daily lifestyle? 1   2   3   4   5

Spiritual Enlightenment

Light of body,
light of mind,
enlightened spirit
is intertwined

Our star, who art within,
Radiance be thy name;
Thy queendom shines,
Thy will be love,
in mind as you are in body.

Give us this light, our daily wow,
and relish our sass and brilliance;
As we dance and follow your siren song,
lead us not into dullsville
but deliver us to succulent joy.

Blissed be.

Alright, so you know the basics of good fuel for your sacred body, and you're geared up with excellent Attitude to approach The Goddess DIET with. Now it's time for the big mama of all heart and mind-shifts: connecting with 'goddess' – aka, *You*.

It is vital that you see and accept yourself as goddess in order to succeed in your mission. You can work out endlessly, starve yourself skinny, stuff yourself fat, envy the glamorous celebrities, but none of these pursuits will bring you satisfaction on their own accord. The key to satisfaction lies within your capacity for self-love. And the key to self-love, in turn, lies within your willingness to embrace your authentic Self: your inner goddess.

Being 'Goddess'

Being goddess doesn't mean being put on a pedestal and worshipped. It's about being the master of your physical, transitional, intuitive, emotional, creative, mental and spiritual well-being. A woman who is connected with her inner goddess is one who truly loves every aspect of herself in all senses. She never concedes her values, and chooses only to honour that which is right for her and for the greatest good of all. Her divine spark is turned *on*.

Some women love being inspired by one archetypal goddess or a specific cultural matriarch to guide them, while others like to work with various goddess energies at different stages of their life (or with different moon phases and so on). Every journey is personal and unique.

After many years of living through all sorts of highs and lows, I have come up with seven key elements that gauge a self-actualised goddess – that is, a woman who is able to transcend inhibitive social expectations or perceived behavioural requirements and instead act in a way that is right for her. It is my intention that once you have completed The Goddess DIET, you will be able to say "Yes, this is me," to each of these statements.

The 7 Gauges of a Self-Actualised Goddess

A self-actualised goddess is a woman who...

1. Celebrates her physical body and her connection to family, humanity, Mother Earth and all her gifts;

2. Is comfortable with infinite abundance, emotional flow and creative freedom;

3. Is proud of her Self and her actions in all her aspects;

4. Fosters mutually fulfilling relationships at all levels;

5. Speaks her truth with diplomacy and shares her lessons with grace;

6. Clearly knows what is right for her, and acts in honour of her innate wisdom and intuition;

7. Revels in her divine purpose/work with gratitude, dignity and generosity.

Each of these gauges is a reflection of the different realms of goddess – some goddesses create, others provide food, some rule, others judge, some offer wisdom, others just wrap us up in their love love love. All aspects of life are represented and reflected in the ancient goddess myths.

Shortly, we'll examine the seven goddess archetypes, how their energy affects your life, and how you can embody their essence in order to see the 'face' of each goddess when you look in the mirror.

But first, read up on the following Intentional Empowerment Tools to enhance your journey to goddess.

Empowerment Tools For Your Spirit

As wonderful as it is to attune your thoughts and attitude to being goddess, sometimes during the course of a busy day, you just need a trigger or a physical object to help realign your focus. Distractions happen, after all. They're natural. So have something ready to use as a power tool for daily use – in your pocket, on your person, in your surrounds, on your wall, in your handbag, or even if it comes to your attention by happenchance, whatever the object is, think of it as your power tool for success.

As hands-on tools are so helpful to people in healing and change, here is a list of additional Intentional Empowerment Tools[38] that you may decide to work with to enhance your journey. Only work with tools that you resonate with, and never rely on any tool to resolve a situation without your willingness to heal or grow at a deep soulular level.

Colours

Natural light (which includes the seven colours of the spectrum) is required for the healthy function of human cells. Filtering natural light through your eyes stimulates your pituary gland, which in turn releases hormones correlating with the organ of the same frequency. This is the science of syntonics and forms the basis of Chromotherapy.

Colours, therefore, are known to resonate with your aura and persona to heighten, lower or balance mood. Surrounding yourself with appropriate colours assists you to respond to situations from an empowered space. Colour therapy can entail the use of gemstones, candles, crystal prisms, tinted eye-glasses, coloured lights, coloured waters, art and mandalas, guided meditation, clothing and makeup.

Essential Oils

Humans have the capability to distinguish 10,000 different smells which all affect our system in three ways – pharmacologically (interacting with the body's chemistry), physiologically (producing a stimulating or sedating effect), and psychologically (prompting emotional responses, often through memory). Aroma-therapy works on our sense of smell and by absorption into the bloodstream. Smells enter the nose where olfactory receptors transport them to the limbic system – the part of the brain that controls our moods, emotions, memory, instinct and learning. Certain smells can prompt memories and unlock emotions thereby bringing subconsciously blocked energy to the surface.

If essential oils sing to you as a tool for healing, please make sure you only use pure oils (avoid 'fragrant' oils as they are synthetic), and seek medical advice before 'playing' with pure essential oils.

Vibrational Essences

Vibrational essences (also referred to as flower remedies) are defined by the World Wide Essence Society (WWES[39]) as "...one of the many ways the natural world offers us to create or maintain health. They contain the energy (also called vital force, life force, chi, or prana) of the flower, gem, place, animal, etc. from which they are made."

Dr Edward Bach first discovered flower essences in the 1930s. He documented the energetic imprints of their life force and their unique abilities to address emotional and mental aspects of wellness based on the homeopathic principle of 'like cures like'. Many other types of vibrational essences have been created since then, that embrace other sources of vibration: gemstones, animals, environment, light, healing energies and intention. The

Goddess-ence vibrational essences, for example, were made with a wide range of source energy including affirmations and days of the week! No matter what the source of vibration, all remedies are intended to remove negative thought patterns, harmonise energy flow, release past traumas, remind us of wisdom we already know, and support us in growing with trust and peace of mind.

Gemstones

Formed over eons, often at high pressure within the earth, gemstones embody intense concentrations of energy. The subsequent energetic and physical properties of gemstones resonate with different parts of the body's energy fields (depending on their origin).

They also have different therapeutic properties depending on their size, shape, exact composition and even the skill of the person holding it. Proper selection, shaping and use transforms them into healing tools. Many healers will tell you the ideal shape for a therapeutic gem is the sphere, but if you are working with a healer whose advice you trust, go with your intuition and do what's right for you.

Sound

In quantum physics we can see that our bodies are made up of atoms and electrons that are in a constant state of oscillation. When they are hit by sound waves, they resonate with the energy of each tone or 'shape' of the sound. Our voice connects our cognitive self to the physical world. Singing, chanting and toning are three ways to get energy flowing through your body. Likewise, sound waves coming into the body (not necessarily through your ears!) help massage your physical and auric bodies, giving you a sense that all is well. During The DIET, enjoy finding a personal theme song each day.

Affirmations

Yes, yes, I'm on about those affirmations again. That's because they're sooooo important for putting yourself in the position of success. They are an invaluable tool for training yourself to think and behave in healthier ways. It's up to you whether you try one of the suggested affirmations each day, whether you make your own, or whether you start out with one from the start and stick with the entire way through.

Grooming

Paying attention to your hair, fingernails, teeth, breath, body hair, moisturising, make-up and perfume is all a part of successful grooming. I'm not saying you have to dress up and make-up every day to be beautiful. Rather, choosing clothes to suit your shape, brushing your teeth and shaving your legs are all acts of self-love. Whether you shave or not; apply make-up or prefer *au naturale*; wear tailored suits or flowing gowns; it doesn't matter... what does matter is that you dress with intention and be conscious about how you present yourself. Taking care of your body and presenting it as healthy is caring about the goddess within. In other words, *embody* the goddess to be *empowered* and *enlightened* in mind, body and spirit.

When you practice respect for your body and your image, it naturally attracts respect from others. As well as making you *look* good in the mirror, proper grooming makes you *feel* good about yourself too. When you feel good, the shift in your attitude is practically tangible. It's easy to walk taller, speak with more confidence and act with more grace. Take note as the Universe sends you more blessings to help you succeed – career gals get pay rises, students win their debates, athletes win more races and mothers get more hugs. Yay for all of this!

Yoga and Movement

The suggested yoga poses in this book come from Natalie
Maisel, a yoga teacher, moon mistress and workshop
leader based in California. Natalie is inspired by goddess
energy in certain yoga positions and associated ritual and
affirmations, which she shares via her website[40]. I love
Natalie's work because she actively and reverently
teaches that yoga is a wonderful practice for helping
women to see themselves as the goddesses they are and
were created to be.

On a physical level, yoga is wonderful for promoting
health because "the asanas, or postures, are beneficial for
every Goddess-y part of you to lengthen your muscles,
increase bone density, cultivate flexibility, encourage
toxin elimination, promote blood flow and circulation,
open the joints, release stale, stuck energy and emotions,
and to cleanse and detoxify your organs."

It also helps on an emotional and spiritual level because
"… the pranayama, breath techniques, will heighten your
Goddess-y awareness of yourself and bring the optimum
amount of oxygen into your body, also releasing carbon
dioxide back into the world to sustain the green life,"
says Natalie.

"Breath is life," she says. "Practising simple breathing
exercises brings your mind, body and emotions into
balance and calms the nervous system within moments."

Daily life brings with it the normal everyday challenges
and triumphs, but "… yoga helps to restore each women
to her supreme glory and recognition of herself. Allow
this ancient practice to transform your life on every level:
physical, mental and emotional," recommends Natalie.

If you're unfamiliar with yoga, please seek professional
assistance to reap the benefits of proper practice.

Using the Tools in The Goddess DIET

During the course of The Goddess DIET, imagine putting on each goddess 'face' once a week over the 21 days. Whilst in this mindset you can then mentally and physically work on each life aspect using each goddess' archetypal energy in conjunction with any (or all) of the tools I've just outlined. Each time you step into a goddess archetype, you are using her story and life lessons as an Intentional Empowerment Tool.

Each goddess archetype resonates exceptionally well with the energy of a particular weekday. It is **not** essential that you work with the archetype energy on a particular day, but going this extra mile adds intensity to your intention. The warrior queen, for example, resonates with Sunday – a day named after the most powerful star in our Universe. Therefore, on each of the three Sundays during The DIET you may choose to focus on being a warrior queen, and conquering issues such as security, sexuality, your connection with family, friends and humanity, and so forth. But if you wake up one day needing to focus on your self-preservation as a matter of urgency, don't wait until Sunday – just spend that day (or a three-day block, or a week, or however long) dealing with that issue.

Here is just a sneak peak of what to expect for each day:

- The ideal day to embrace your warrior queen is a Sunday. You may dedicate the three Sundays throughout The DIET to celebrating your physical body and your connection to your physical world. Your key life aspect is **security** and your focus is on self-preservation.

- On Mondays, you may embody your magical muse. Become more comfortable with infinite abundance, emotional flow, transitional well-being and creative freedom. Your key life aspect as a magical muse is **creativity**. Focus on what brings you self-gratification.

- Tuesday is a great day to shine as a daring diva. Develop your intuitive wisdom, pride yourself in all your aspects, and make choices that honour your needs. Your key life aspect on this day is **power**. Focus on developing your self-definition.

- On Wednesdays, you may welcome your primordial mother. Energised by this 'mother lode' of love, gain a better understanding of how to foster mutually fulfilling relationships at all levels. Your key life aspect while wearing this 'face' is **love**. Focus on developing your self-acceptance.

- On Thursdays, love your journey with your natural healer within. Begin to relish speaking your truth with diplomacy, and sharing your insights with grace. Your key life aspect on this day is **truth**. Focus on developing your self-expression.

- On Fridays, welcome your sacred sage. It will become increasingly clear to you what is right for you. Enjoy acting in honour of your innate wisdom and intuition. Your key life aspect on this day is **trust**. Focus on developing your self-reflection.

- And, on Saturdays, be uplifted with your high priestess. Revel in your divine purpose and work with gratitude, dignity and generosity. Your key life aspect as a high priestess is joy. Focus on developing your self-knowledge.

Don't worry if this is sounding like too much to remember. There are lots of prompts in Part 3 of this book (and even more in *The Goddess DIET Companion*) to raise your consciousness throughout the process. So relax, and take each day at a time to journey with pleasure.

The 7 Faces of Goddess

It's no secret that women have many faces. In just one day you can be Ms Professional at work; partner, cook, entertainer, counsellor, scheduler and carer at home; taxi driver, nurse, earth mother and teacher for the kids; socialite and confidant with friends; and Princess MeMe when you go bar-hopping. Looking to the ancient goddesses as role models is one way to handle every situation with your integrity intact.

The goddesses also have many faces. During the DIET you will be donning the 'face' of each archetype in order to become conscious of how her energy manifests in you, and so you can recognise her in the mirror. You will have 'a-ha' moments when realise the parallels between each archetype' challenges and victories, with those in your own life as a modern woman. You will experience how empowering it is to embody each archetype as a tool for holistic well-being. And you will feel invincible when you realise these tools are very easy to use in everyday life – simply say, "I am (archetype)," and respond to each situation accordingly from that space. The seven faces of goddess are:

Goddess Aspect	Domain
Warrior Queen	Self-preservation / security
Magical Muse	Self-gratification / creativity
Daring Diva	Self-definition/ power
Primordial Mother	Self-acceptance / love
Natural Healer	Self-expression / truth
Sacred Sage	Self-reflection / trust
High Priestess	Self-knowledge / joy

Warrior Queen: Self-Preservation / Security

History is saturated with the deeds, ingenuity and strength of warrior queens: Greek goddess Athena, Celtic queen Bodicea, Egyptian pharaoh-queen Hatshepsut, Elizabeth I, Marie Antoinette... the list is as endless as it is inspirational. All these queens share common attributes of resilience, poise, self-assurance and a dynamic presence.

Warrior queens have unshakeable trust in their abilities to lead. Without hesitation they are prepared to stand up for their rights and the rights of others who rely on them for security. They forge ahead despite (or because of) obstacles. They carve their own path and lead by example. They stay balanced in times or duress, and connected to their traditions and sources of inspiration whether they be at war or in peace. They are in tune with their physical body and are deeply connected with Mother Earth and humanity.

Being warrior queen is about being in tune with your physical body, and being able to respond to threatening situations rationally and calmly. Don't assume that 'warrior' only implies violence or force – well chosen words can be as influential and as satisfying as swinging a sword in any argument or cause.

It means you can be conscious of others' moods and needs and stay balanced in times of duress; trust your instinct and act with the confidence that comes from a deeply rooted connection with earth; manifest a dynamic presence by walking confidently on your path; and feel secure by keeping your feet firmly on the ground. It also means fostering the physical health and social affinity of your family, friends, community and Mother Earth in equal measure.

Archetypal Goddesses that are Warrior Queens

Greek goddess of love and fertility, fire and productivity, war and victory and sexual prowess, **Astarte** exemplifies the spirit that drives us to success, both in achieving goals and surviving life's battles.

Hindu goddess of destruction, **Kali** rips the carpet from under your feet and turns your life upside-down, but only so that you can find your true life path. She also helps you get rid of your attachment to excess baggage.

Freja is the Nordic goddess of love and war. The cycle of life and death is inevitable, so her lesson is: celebrate the beginning and the end (which is really the beginning again), and be passionate about everything in between.

She may be known as the goddess of summer flowers, the Queen of May and a graceful faery spirit, but Welsh goddess **Cordelia** is no sissy. She had the respect of her father's kingdom for her light-filled energy and grace under pressure. Leading by example, she teaches us to stand firm with dignity and quiet determination.

If it's a tigress mother you're looking for, embrace the Celtic warrior queen, **Bodicea**. Legend has it that she killed an entire army to avenge the rape of her daughters. Thus, she exemplifies focussed and champion energy.

Artemis is the moon goddess whose gift of strength helps you say no to forces that inhibit you. You are a powerful being able to bring an end to destructive forces in order to start afresh.

Greek goddess of courage, **Athena** guarded the ancient city of Athens and saved it from destruction. Athena-gals are uncannily resourceful and know how to kick butt.

More information about goddesses: Goddess.com.au

Manifest your Warrior Queen

The best day for manifesting your warrior queen is on a Sunday. Sunday is named in honour of the sun – the centre of our Solar system, source of light and sustainer of life. It is linked with the base chakra – the auric energy field located at the bottom of your spine. Just as the planets revolve around the sun, our base chakra acts like an anchor to all the aspects of our life and connects us with the physical plane. It fires our survival instincts, and in grounding us, forms the basis of our security, whether that security be in terms of employment, income, moral or physiological, family-based or health related.

When you look in the mirror, see determination on your face, strength along your spine and leadership in your stance. Your feet should be firmly planted on the floor, and if it helps you feel more stable, bend your knees slightly. Your body language is saying, "I am invincible. I am present. I am perfectly grounded and secure." If it helps, visualise yourself carrying Athena's sword.

Natalie Maisel recommends the Athena posture (Warrior II) to manifest this archetypal energy.

"Empower yourself by adopting Athena pose," she says. "Athena was known as the Goddess who is nobody's fool! She refused to be a girly girl, but chose a life as a true wild woman. She could match any man's game and carried herself with dignity and inner power. Stand tall and courageous with your unerring arrow aimed at your goal. You are a Goddess of strength, wildness and vision. As you hold your posture, call on Athena with this chant, *Conceive it, believe it, take aim to achieve it, let go to Athena, prepare to receive it"*

Support yourself during the day with a selection of tools, listed herewith.

Colour Surround yourself in red to raise energy levels, willpower and enthusiasm. It gives you greater confidence to stride boldly on your path, and, happily, it promotes lustier sex. Red also protects you from negative influences, feelings and anxieties.

Essential Oils Burn oils such as ginger to boost self-confidence. Blend ginger with lavender, patchouli and palmarosa for their calming and balancing properties, and grapefruit white to energise your willpower.

Gemstones Place red stones in your underwear drawer where they can energise items worn against your base chakra. Or add a new dimension to 'stonewash jeans' and carry stones in your jeans pockets. Garnet aids commitment and balances libido; Bloodstone helps you accept change; Tourmaline grounds spiritual energy; and Smoky Quartz fortifies resolve.

Sound Play crystal bowls and bells in the tone of C. Stomp in time to earthenware drums. If you'd prefer to dance along with some music, go for soul, gospel and anything with a fat base guitar.

Affirmations I am grounded and secure
My path reveals itself to me
I have the energy to do all I want
I am Warrior Woman, hear me roar!
The more I move, the more energy I have
Earth is my mother and I am home
Conceive it, believe it, take aim to achieve it,
let go to Athena, prepare to receive it

Magical Muse: Self-Gratification / Creativity

Magical muses are the goddesses that rule over creativity, self-gratification, abundance and the feminine divine: Ishtar, Venus, Aphrodite, and the nine daughters of the Greek goddess Mnemosyne… they show us how to creatively, emotionally and sexually connect with others with respect and fluidity.

The magical muse is able to accept change gracefully. She openly and readily releases any need to control external forces. She can step into the flow of life whilst maintaining her sense of purpose. She has a magnetic aura and her body confidence is alluring and sensual. As such, she loves words like succulent, curvaceous, juicy and divine.

In the aspect of abundance, the magical muse naturally attracts that which is exactly right for her. She asks for what she deserves and gives herself permission to receive it. She relishes beauty, embodies grace and attracts both attributes with ease. She teaches us that a poverty consciousness only serves to deny you what you deserve. Abundance is good, (greed is not), whether it be material, esoteric, emotional or otherwise. Ask for what you want and deserve, and give yourself permission to receive it.

Optimists and free thinkers are able to utilise fluctuating energies and live life to the max. They can make meaningful friendships with others through creativity, emotional tolerance and sensuality. By putting on the face of the magical muse, we can learn to accept change gracefully, release anxieties and forgive past hurts. And, we are able to step into creative flow like never before – words, ideas, concepts, colours, sparkles and wonder simply, flows effortlessly. As we surrender to the flow, we are able to receive all these gifts back in equal measure.

Archetypal Goddesses that are Magical Muses

One goddess that acts as role model in the realm of magical muse is the patroness of belly-dancers, **Ishtar**. She is the Babylonian goddess of love and sensuality and inspires lovers every-where to connect with the feminine divine. Under her influence, women can embrace the true essence of what it means to be woman – graceful, feline and sensual.

West African, Brazilian and Afro-Caribbean goddess **Yemaya** is Mother Water, orisha of the oceans. She is mother love; a deep ocean of comfort for those in need.

Baubo, the ancient Grecian goddess, is one of many wild goddesses of sacred sexuality. A crone goddess with irreverent joy and liberation towards sexuality, she reminds us to relish sex, love, and above all, laughter.

Earth Mother, **Ceres** represents the cycles we experience as part of human nature, and allows us to accept the ebbs and flows graciously. She empowers us to find our centre and gently go with the flow.

Tyche is the Greek goddess of fortune who rules your degree of life and luck. Tyche's dice will roll in your favour when you help others improve their fortune.

Likewise, **Sri Laxmi** is the goddess of good fortune, ability and diligence. Wealth is the manifestation of these attributes when they are in flow.

Regardless of your shape or size, **Aphrodite** is here to inspire a charming and magnetic charisma. This Greek goddess of love and beauty drove every god wild with desire, which only served to fuel her flirtatious nature. She is a role model for pure sensuality and magnetism.

More information about goddesses: Goddess.com.au

Manifest your Magical Muse

The best day for manifesting your magical muse is on a Monday. The correlation between Monday's namesake, the moon, and women is intrinsically linked. Feminine cycles reflect the moon's journey, just as cycles ebb and flow through the phases of new, emerging, full and waning energies. It is consequently the seat of our shifting moods and emotions.

These are energies that are linked with the sacral chakra, located below the navel. Creativity is heightened when this sacral chakra is awakened. Balancing this aspect of your life enables you to accept responsibility for your own choices and desires, accept change gracefully, release anxieties and past hurts, and let the depth of your feelings show.

When you look in the mirror, connect with your magical muse by relaxing your stance and accentuating your curves. Get creative! Cup your belly or frame it with your hands. Soften your body lines and shimmy!

As for a yoga pose, Natalie recommends the Aphrodite posture (Garland pose / deep squat) with your hands on your sacral chakra.

"Aphrodite is the Goddess of pleasure and sensuality," says Natalie. "She never met a man she didn't like. Her womanly wiles were enough to seduce any potential lover! She is a true diva – a Goddess who isn't afraid to allure, seduce and satiate. Call on Aphrodite to rekindle your passion for yourself, your lover or life in general.

As you hold your posture, call on Aphrodite with this chant, *Aphrodite, Aphrodite, come to me, fill me with passion and creativity.*"

Colour   Add orange to your life to become more
                    enthusiastic and active about a project; to
                    increase creative urges and flow; to spice
                    things up if you're in a rut; and as relief
                    from getting too serious about life.

Essential Oils Ylang ylang is used for its anti-depressant
                    qualities. To reach the centre of your
                    creativity and personal power, sweet
                    orange is used along with grapefruit
                    white to relieve anxiety and patchouli for
                    its calming effect.

Gemstones   Orange gemstones These can also be
                    carried in your jeans pockets against your
                    sacral chakra. Carnelian restores vitality
                    and promotes trust in nature's cycles;
                    Citrine opens intuition and promotes
                    creativity and abundance; Brown Jasper is
                    connected with the earth and detoxifies
                    the body's organs.

Sound   Swirl and swing your hips in time to
                    hypnotic trances and belly-dancing music.
                    Listen to music or play crystal bowls in
                    the tone of D, chant the sacred vowel BA.

Affirmations   My creativity flows easily
                    I am woman – sexy and wise
                    I am woman – hear me purrrrr
                    I am the luckiest woman on earth
                    I relinquish control to my Higher Power
                    I am wild, succulent, and my divine spark
                    is absolutely *on*
                    I have an abundance of time, health,
                    happiness and wealth
                    *Aphrodite, Aphrodite, come to me, fill me with
                    passion and creativity*

Daring Diva: Self-Definition / Power

Any goddess or patroness that inspires you to step into your own personal power is a daring diva: the Greek maiden Persephone, volcano goddess Pele and moon goddess Diana are just a few role models whose stories we can be inspired by.

A daring diva is able to present her stunning and glorious Self to the world whether the world likes it or not! She is absolutely *real* whether she is performing on stage in the lead role, supporting from back stage or simply content to be relaxing in the audience. She rises above superficiality and allows her inner wisdom to be her guiding force in decision-making and her actions. She is intrinsically connected to her intuitive Self and she is readily able to marshal her personal power for her highest good. She knows that anxiety and 'butterflies' that sit in her belly is simply her inner tigress preparing her for success.

In short, a daring diva is the leading lady in her own life. Daring divas have learned uncompromising strength, compassion and justice. They have mastered self-ownership, and understand they are responsible for their own actions, how they react to others, and for presenting their authentic Self to the world.

These goddesses encourage you to delve deeper than the superficial exterior that we have been conditioned to develop and present.

To become a daring diva, spend time on self-definition. Work out who you are, who you want to be, and then honour the true you in the image you present to everyone you meet. Work with a relevant archetypal goddess who encompasses daring diva energy.

Archetypal Goddesses that are Daring Divas

Hawaiian volcano goddess, **Pele** houses her boiling energy in her belly. When it all gets too much, she purges this bubbling mass of fiery energy in spectacular style. She calms down again to find she has changed her environment forever (this is not always a bad thing!)

Depicted in art as lusciously curvy, the Roman goddess **Venus** fully owns her Rubenesque shape and feminine divine. She rules over your sense of style and your appreciation for acts of love, pleasure and romance.

Oya is the African goddess storms, tempests and rain. Her winds of change sweep away the old in order to prepare for the new. She wreaks destruction so that you can find and prepare for underlying calm.

Diana's short skirt is not for attracting male attention, but is more a symbol of freedom. This Roman goddess of nature remains free to leap through the forests and touch the sky with her outstretched fingers.

Sumerian goddess **Lilith** is honoured for her wisdom, freedom, courage, playfulness and sexuality. Portrayed as a demon by frustrated priests, she is a pioneer in equality between the sexes by remaining true to feminine wisdom.

The namesake for month of May, **Maia** is remembered as the goddess of spring and rebirth. She makes the lush green grass and the fragrant flowers grow again.

Persephone spent her time between being Maiden of Spring and Queen of Darkness, proving that it is entirely possible to stand wholly in your power no matter what the circumstances. She is a role model in accepting both your light and shadow sides. Her lesson is that you can be equally as powerful in either space.

More information about goddesses: Goddess.com.au

Manifest your Daring Diva

The best day for manifesting your daring diva is on a Tuesday, the day named after the planet Mars. Being the planet representing war and conflict, Tuesday is therefore the perfect day to think about all things associated with courage, action, initiative and daring.

Tuesday is also related to the solar plexus chakra, nick-named the power chakra. It rules our personal power, fear, autonomy and metabolism. When in balance, this life aspect brings us magnetic energy, effectiveness, spontaneity, and a healthy sense of Self.

When looking in the mirror, look within. Gaze into your eyes and spend time working out who you are, who you want to be, and then honouring the authentic You in your choices and behaviour. Modify your posture to reflect this connection with your power. It could be a warrior stance or a butterfly in flight to represent your light side, or perhaps your pose is initially 'nausea' or a wounded child to represent your shadow side. Either way, you'll be able to reveal your daring diva naturally by being completely honest with yourself.

Natalie recommends the Nile Goddess posture (Utkatasana / fierce pose) and says, "Be yourself!"

Yes! "Simply, powerfully, authentically YOU. Nothing to hide behind, nothing to squirm from, nothing to be afraid of. You are the Egyptian Nile River Goddess rising high above worldly concerns and drama. As you assume the Nile Goddess posture, notice how your hands are like the waxing and waning moons – a perfect representation of sacred balance. Consciously draw in what you choose, and release what no longer works. Maintain this pose as you recite, *"the Nile is rising, the Nile is falling, I bring in, and I let go."*

Colour   Yellow helps achieve greater clarity in
                      your decision-making, it increases
                      concentration when studying for exams or
                      preparing for your annual job review, it
                      improves digestion and appetite, and it
                      brings some sunshine on cloudy days.

Essential Oils Lemongrass and eucalyptus are used to
                      cleanse and decongest the chakra ready
                      for the energies of rosewood, peppermint
                      and bergamot to uplift the senses, and
                      lime and lemon myrtle to promote clarity
                      and confidence.

Gemstones   Carry or wear yellow gemstones to
                      promote your unique style. They also
                      improve your ability and willingness to
                      listen to your intuition. Amber promotes
                      drive to achieve goals; Tiger Eye promotes
                      integrity and intention; Yellow Jade boosts
                      determination and helps eliminate waste.

Sound   Sing aloud to any song that describes or
                      resonates with who you are or who you
                      want to be. Play crystal bowls in the tone
                      of E, and chant the sacred vowel of YM.

Affirmations I am me!
                      I am protected and priceless
                      Others are inspired by my energy
                      I am the embodiment of sunshine
                      I deserve to be treated with respect
                      I am valuable, self-confident and strong
                      I'm my own tigress mother and superstar
                      I claim my personal power, hear me roar!
                      *The Nile is rising, the Nile is falling, I bring
                      in, and I let go*

Primordial Mother: Self-Acceptance / Love

Mother love is arguably the strongest, sweetest, most enduring love of all. Kwan Yin, White Tara, Mary and Demeter are just some role models who exemplify mother love in their unconditional love for their children.

The primordial mother embodies love, compassion and trust. All these attributes are a two-way street for her – as happily as she gives these gifts to others, she receives them back unto herself. She never, ever allows herself to accept second best because she knows that in order to shower love upon others she must be ready to accept it in equal measure. The primordial mother revels in her self-respect, self-love and self-appreciation. Her inner child is a reflection of her perfection. Her heart is open and willing to trust. She thinks love; she *is* love.

The primordial mother never ignores her birthright of love and respect. She knows that if she doesn't personify both self-love and self*less* love easily, she can't expect others to behave with self-respect either. Furthermore, she knows that by letting others treat her badly, she is telling her authentic self that she does not deserve better. Therefore, she behaves in accordance with the three G-Forces of love: Grace, Generosity and Gratitude.

When we break down walls made of fear, guilt and mistrust, we invite in joy, reciprocated love and uplifting light. In releasing the three Heartbreak-Rs (Regrets, Reproach and Retribution), primordial mothers teach us how to rally our self-respect. We become role models for happiness and inspiration to others, fostering mutual love and harmony. Work with these life aspects and goddesses so that you can inspire others to whoop with delight: "I'll have what she's having!"

Archetypal Goddesses that are Primordial Mothers

Chinese mother of compassion, **Kwan Yin** is a source of comfort and peace. Her values are about balance, sharing, harmony, co-operation and partnership; she demonstrates highly tuned tolerance and acceptance.

Demeter's search for her lost daughter became all-consuming to the detriment of her people's crops and harvests. Her perseverance and determination paid off as she successfully negotiated the return of Persephone.

No matter what time of the year, earth mother **Gaia** nourishes you with her produce and provides you with her inherent wisdom of nature, animals and elements. To the Romans she was the greatest mother of all.

With her third eye and eyes in each hand and foot, Tibetan goddess **Tara** sees beyond the mortal veil into eternity. She reminds us that all things pass and each moment is perfect.

Hestia represents purity, sincerity, sanctity and safety. She was the keeper of the sacred fire on Mount Olympus, and as such, came to symbolise an uncomplicated, enriching and contented life.

Prepared to go to any lengths to protect her relationship with her husband, Roman goddess **Juno** gives us the energy to fight for the elements we want and deserve in a relationship.

If home is where the heart is, call on the Roman goddess of household abundance and well-being, **Vesta**. She energises the home with a welcoming energy for bountiful, healthy food and comfort.

More information about goddesses: Goddess.com.au

Manifest your Primordial Mother

The best day for manifesting primordial mother is on a Wednesday. This is the day associated with the heart chakra, the home of the greatest force in the Universe – love. Located in the middle of the upper and lower chakras it is the balance of opposites in the psyche: mind and body, yin and yang. Likewise, Wednesday is the middle of the week. It is named after Mercury which rules over intellect, versatility, healing and mediation.

When you look in the mirror with your primordial mother face on, see love, love, love in your reflection. Let warmth shine from your eyes, and forgiveness and self-love from your heart. Notice how your primordial mother manifests – it could be a 'look' of admiration, a nod of approval, or a generous smile. If you have trouble getting started with shining mother love for your Self, imagine you are looking at your child. What happens to your body and your attitude? Give yourself a big mother-of-all-hugs when you are able to bask in your perfection.

Natalie recommends the Mother Mary posture (seated baby cradle) to further open this energetic awareness.

"How much can you love yourself today? How much can you love another?" she prompts. "Know that there is no limit on the amount of love you can give and receive. As you practice Mother Mary pose, imagine that you are holding yourself as a small child in your own arms. Rock this baby that is you. Feel the love emanating from your heart centre as you breathe. Mother Mary Goddess is considered the mother of eternal love. Invoke her energy as you gaze lovingly and inwardly at yourself. Let her powerful radiance fill you with peace and love that knows no bounds. Chant a sweet lullaby as you hold your pose with this affirmation: *"I am loved, I am cradled, I am adored."*

Colour	Green is the colour of nature, healing, growth, safety and new beginnings. Pink increases kindness, acceptance and trust. Use it to accept help, find new levels of calmness and reduce fears of intimacy.
Essential Oils	Sweet orange reduces anxiety, lemon (clarity), geranium bourbon and chamomile balances mood swings, grapefruit white stimulates energy flow, and jasmine absolute is an aphrodisiac that brings optimism and balance.
Gemstones	Green gemstones promote prosperity, balance and fertility. Pink stones promote love, self-worth and trust. Wear these stones on a chain long enough so they can rest near your heart. Rose quartz promotes unconditional love and inner healing; green tourmaline helps with patience and deeper bonds with others; and emerald is a symbol of patience and abiding joy.
Sound	Play any song that pulls on the heartstrings. Love songs open you to possibilities, as do sing-alongs with friends. Play music in the tone of F and chant the sacred vowel HA.
Affirmations	I think love, I am love I live in perfect love and trust Self-acceptance brings me joy Love lifts me up where I belong ;-) I am worthy of incredible happiness Forgiveness is healthy and comes easily My heart is open to loving relationships *I am loved, I am cradled, I am adored*

Natural Healer: Self-Expression / Truth

Words have the power to hurt as well as to heal. In order to use words wisely, call on one of the many goddesses who rule over self-expression and healing: the Irish queen Dana, the islander goddess Hina, Hindu goddess of prosperity Sri Laxmi, or the Welsh goddess Rhiannon.

The natural healer is able to choose her words wisely to facilitate understanding. Her shared insights are precise, astute and relevant. She is able to seek and accept help, ask for abundance for her highest good, and make her point without aggression. She understands that her expressions manifest in exactly the way she describes. She aids effective communication between the genders, the young and the old, the experienced and the novice. When she speaks, she is heard. Just as easily, when others speak, she listens. She is often clairaudient in that she senses or hears (and heeds) Angels and other spiritual beings.

There are many goddesses who rule over the domain of self-expression. They teach us how to ask for things for our highest good, and how our expressions manifest in exactly the way we describe. Draw on the examples of the natural healers to implement the Law of Attraction and the Law of Benevolence. Remember your remedial talents from this life and others. Revert to natural and gentle ways of healing rifts and treating wounds. Only make promises you can keep. Banish stagnancy, bring in creative instinct and expression. Understand that plain sailing does not a master sailor make.

Consider these goddesses your role models as you work with the life aspect resonating with you now.

Archetypal Goddesses that are Natural Healers

Dana is the mother goddess of the Irish faery people, the Tuatha Dé Danann (too-ha-day-dah-nan). They were skilled in art, poetry and magic, and ruled Ireland until they were overrun and driven to live in faery mounds. Though Christian monks recorded many Irish legends, sadly there are no recorded stories of Dana. Evidently her latent message is to tell your story before it is too late!

Goddess **Fortuna** promises riches and abundance, and nurtures our individual destinies through the ups and downs of the life cycle. She rewards those with joyful intentions with success and prosperity.

Wise and magical Welsh goddess of the moon, **Rhiannon** hears our wishes and guides us on the path of inspiration – but only if we learn how to ask.

Greek goddess **Iambe** is credited with the poetry style of iambic pentameter (think of Shakespeare verse). She relishes laughter, merriment and mirth to restore your connection to your authentic self.

Champion of words and ideas, **Hina** (associated with Tahiti, Hawaiian, and Pacific Island cultures) represents meaningful communication between goddess sisters, and facilitates the sharing of truth between women and men.

Just as water ebbs and flows, the Nigerian goddess **Oshun** teaches us to go with the flow of our instincts in order to find calmer waters.

If you have a nasty habit of saying "it's too hard," work with the Greek goddess **Athena**. Just as she guarded the ancient city of Athens and saved it from destruction, draw on her courage to fight your own battles too.

More information about goddesses: Goddess.com.au

Manifest your Natural Healer

Thursday is a fabulous day for working with natural healer energy as it is named after Jupiter, the planet that signifies expansion and growth. Jupiter represents strong morals, prosperity, maturity, dependability and luck. It takes 12 years for this planet to orbit the sun, but let's hope it can take you less time than that to learn to express what it is you need to say to bring you happiness. Trust and honour higher forces at work within you to keep your throat chakra open and vibrant.

Sit and look into the mirror as though having a conversation with the person in the reflection. Actually have a conversation with that person via ESP. Nod to show you are listening and take note of your gesticulations and posture when you express concerns or joys. Embrace the posture that radiates awareness and understanding.

Natalie loves doing the Goddess Dana (butterfly/baddha konasana) pose to connect with her inner natural healer. She modifies is slightly by putting her hands over her throat chakra.

"Practising Goddess Dana pose will enable you to release pent up, harsh or unsaid words and blocked feelings," she says, and that's a healthy thing.

"Dana was also known as the queen of the fairies, so as you move into this posture, notice how your legs are like the wings of a fairy that will help you fly away, high above old ways of living and being that are no longer useful to you. Hold this posture with both hands placed on your throat area. Make a humming sound that helps to release anything blocked in the throat chakra. As your humming gets louder and stronger, you will sound like a million fairies in flight."

Colours   Unlike emotionally warm colours like red, orange and yellow, light blue influences intellect and logic. Use this colour for harmony and to counteract tension with tact and negotiation. Also use light blue to ease depression ('the blues') and to broaden your perspective of your world.

Essential Oils Vetiver provides a stable base to prepare for new opportunities. Use with cedarwood to decongest the airways. Lemon and cajeput bring clarity and vision, lavender balances your new energy, and frankincense rejuvenates intentions.

Gemstones   Blue gemstones help calm 'troubled waters' with words and actions. Lapis lazuli guards against psychic attack; aquamarine facilitates tolerance; and turquoise enhances earthly and spiritual communication for true soulful expression. Wear these stones around your neck.

Sound   Sing your favourite songs at the top of your voice. Harmonise with your children and teach them how to 'let it all out'. Be like Liza Minelli and belt out cabaret, show tunes, freedom songs and gospel music. Play crystal bowls in the tone of G and chant the sacred vowel of RE.

Affirmations   I am safe to speak my truth
                   I invite new choices into my life
                   My inner child is seen and heard
                   My words flow with ease and grace
                   I am full of ideas and able to express them
                   I find the right words at the right time

Sacred Sage: Self-Reflection / Trust

"Know thyself," says Shakespeare, as do the many goddesses who rule over the domain of self-reflection: the Egyptian goddess Isis, the Celtic goddess Brigid and the wise woman, Hecate. They teach us to trust our innate wisdom and to allow that wisdom be our guide.

The sacred sage is readily and easily able to move on from petty issues. She opens her vision to see alternative views (and viewpoints). She lives in a state of clarity because she is able to release negative elements that no longer serve her: self-judgement, self-criticism, self-scorn. She regularly simplifies her life, both physically and mentally, and enjoys the liberation that comes with being in a state of *simplicitas*. She has regular bursts of epiphany, relishes symbolism, and is grateful for the many miracles that present themselves to her every day.

She is often the first person people come to for advice. Her ability to think outside the square and offer advice with impartiality means she is a wonderful source of common sense. She knows that trivial worries are simply a distraction mechanism to keep her from what it is she really needs to see. Getting over the petty stuff is easy for the sacred sage because she knows that seeing the bigger picture is a far better outlook.

The sacred sage likes to stay sharp and up to date with current affairs. She keeps her wits about her by using her brain. She partakes in left- and right-brain activities, lively conversations, adult education and journal-writing. It is often in the process of journalling that she is most able to self-reflect and find solutions by remaining open to divine guidance.

Archetypal Goddesses that are Sacred Sages

Egyptian high priestess **Isis** has a connection with the psychic realm that allows us to cultivate our trust in our own psychic wisdom.

Hathor was the Ancient Queen of Heaven who brings the gift of shape shifting – using Hathor as a role model, we can transform from a coper to a radiant stunwana.

The ancient Slavic goddess **Baba Yaga** is the wild old crone who holds a dark mirror to our souls. It is through examination of our dark sides that we can be reborn.

Celtic goddess of healing, light, inspiration and all skills associated with fire, **Brigid** is the benefactress of inner healing and vital energy.

Inanna's transformational journey into the underworld (through shame, pain and near death), and subsequent emergence bigger'n'better'n'ever, represents the soul's evolution through hardship into glorious renewal.

The Celtic goddess **Epona** and her white mare accompanies the soul on its final journey to the other world. She helps manifest your dreams if you allow her to accompany you on your path.

Greek goddess **Mnemosyne** was originally honoured as the Greek goddess of memory, but is largely known today as the mother of the nine muses of the creative arts. In acknowledging your story, you can easily recognise your full potential as wonderful, sacred, self-fulfilled being.

Life's too short to hide in your cave forever, as the Japanese sun goddess **Amaterasu** found out. She moped in a cave to hide from a harsh situation, but did eventually venture out to share her radiance once again.

More information about goddesses: Goddess.com.au

Manifest your Sacred Sage

Friday is my favourite day of all. It was named after Freja, the Scandinavian goddess of passion, love and war. Her followers envisaged dining with her in the after-life (in Valhalla) thus enhancing their abilities to see beyond the physical realm. Friday, therefore, is the day to open your psychic faculties and understand your life purpose.

On Fridays envisage Freya's passion and harness that energy to explore your highest possibilities to the highest degree for your highest good. Go to your 'happy place', empty your mind of trivial and conditioned thinking, and aim to think bigger, wider and deeper than ever before. Get back to your passion and get your passion back.

When you look in the mirror, pose as though in prayer or meditation, and simply, *be*. It doesn't matter if your eyes are closed or open, but it is important that you are comfortable in the presence of the wise woman gazing back at you from the glass.

Natalie loves doing the Isis posture (Warrior III) to access her inner sacred sage.

"The Egyptian Goddess Isis was the medicine woman of the Nile. She was mid-wife, healer, wife and lover. Her tears over the loss of her husband, Osiris, caused the Nile river to flood. But, Isis was a Goddess who had it together, and knew what she was made of. She taught women to love deeply and strongly and deal with grief by having the greater vision to continue with life and be a beacon of strength to all those who need it," says Natalie.

"As you hold the Isis pose, imagine that you are flying high above pain, loss, betrayal and sadness. See with your greater vision and trust your own process in life's great journey. Chant, *Isis, I see. Isis, I see, the gift life is meant to be*."

Colours	Add indigo to your life to heighten intuition, rise above any ruts, enjoy solitude, or find a solution to a problem.
Essential Oils	Cedarwood atlas unblocks energy flows ready for rosemary, a brain stimulant that promotes clarity, calming lavender, frankincense and lemon for rejuvenation, and basil to assist with decision making in your new space of vision and insight.
Gemstones	Dark blue gemstones help open your sub-conscious and promote trust in your Self. Moonstone facilitates deep appreciation for the cycle of change and lucid dreaming; sodalite opens spiritual perception and is useful in meditation; and dark aquamarine calms the mind and clarifies perception.
Sound	Play meditative music and allow your mind to roam, explore possibilities and find answers 'out of the blue'. Teach your children to sing the alphabet. Challenge your intellect and sing it backwards. Hum along to crystal bowls in the tone of A and chant the sacred vowel of AH.
Affirmations	I trust my intuition Clarity, clarity, clarity I make way for love and light My wisdom is all-encompassing I trust that my body is GORGEOUS Every choice I make is the right one I see the goddess' gifts all around me My divine light ignites the light in others *Isis, I see. Isis, I see, the gift life is meant to be.*

High Priestess: Self-Knowledge / Joy

Call the connection to the realm of bliss what you will,
but there comes a time when everyone seeks a connection
to a higher consciousness or realm. Goddesses that
preside over self-knowledge and cosmic connection
include the Welsh goddess Cerridwen, Egyptian goddess
Nuit, and American Indian weaver of life, Spider Woman.

The high priestess is able to see herself as a minute
organism in the ways of the world, both in the physical
and non-physical planes, in the present and the future.
She is a cosmic traveller, time expander and a sacred
vessel for divine expression. She believes in
disconnecting from the world every now and then in
order to travel to a spaceless, timeless place of all-
knowing. Intuitively and effortlessly, she shares her gifts
of wisdom, understanding and spiritual knowledge.
She knows her calling and honours her destiny. Everyday
matters don't concern her as much as the divine well-
being of all living creatures. She is the gateway to the
answers that lie in the great beyond. Prayer and ritual put
her on a spiritual high that transcends earthly concerns.
She sits in the palm of god and in the heart of goddess.

One of the high priestess' favourite past-times is star-
gazing to remind her she is, at the same time, both
microscopic and infinite. She loves to follow particular
constellations that transit across her sky. During the day
she sees stairways to heaven, omens in the clouds, and
'fingers of Nuit' streaming to earth. Out of all the
archetypes, she is most easily able to interpret messages
from Mother Earth via symbols and animals.

High priestess energy is sourced from the more magical,
cosmic and crone goddesses. Depending on what life
stage you are at, different aspects will appeal.

Archetypal Goddesses that are High Priestesses

Egyptian goddess, **Nuit** is the bridge between heaven and earth. She helps us bond with our planetary family while soaring in her realm of cosmic consciousness. She fosters your skills in astral travelling, following stardust trails, taking moon walks and blissful meditation.

Spider Woman is the Native American great teacher, protector and Mother of all creation. Imparting her sacred wisdom to us as we sleep, she connects all her children through a filament spun from her crown.

Goddess of the moon and the night, **Circe** began life as a mage for hire in order to fund her expensive pursuit of magic. She challenges you to take responsibility for your own actions and life in order to steer your destiny.

Hecate completes the goddess triad of the Maiden, the Matron and the Maven. She walks between the seen and unseen world but resides in neither, carrying a flaming torch to guide you at crossroads.

The dark Welsh goddess, **Cerridwen**, of great wisdom, prophetic foresight, and magical shape-shifting abilities lends us her relentless energy and focus required to achieve our ultimate goals.

Mayan moon goddess **IxChel** wears a serpent on her head representing transformation. Just like the snake, she sheds her winter skin in order to blossom anew into spring to a new and fresh stage in the life cycle.

Bast, or Bastet, is an Egyptian goddess of the sun and Greeks goddess of the moon. She's also the ancestral mother of all cats and thus, the patron of play. She is adept at finding the perfect balance between discipline and fun.

More information about goddesses: Goddess.com.au

Manifest your High Priestess

It is a beautiful thing to celebrate high priestess energy on Saturdays – the day named after Saturn, whose properties are discipline, patience and perseverance. In ancient times it was the furthest planet that could be seen by the naked eye. Its seemingly infinite journey around the Sun connects us to a place of immeasurable time and space, as does the crown chakra which becomes our channel to pure awareness through consciousness.

There are many forms of knowledge – cognitive, emotional, intuitive, learned, to name a few. But 'wisdom' is a whole new level of understanding that transcends the physical plane. When awakened, this chakra brings us such wisdom, knowledge, understanding, spiritual connection, and bliss.

When you look in the mirror, stand with your palms facing upwards and your hands raised towards the source of your divine inspiration. You are the embodiment of joy and bliss. Celebrate this *knowing* and let it show.

Natalie does this by doing practising the Nuit Sky Goddess (baby dancer/Lord Natarajasana) pose.

"Nuit painted the sky and is covered in twinkling stars. Bliss is her middle name and joy is her game!" she says.

"Embody Nuit's cosmic character by practising Nuit Sky Goddess pose and embodying her celestial spirit. As you enter this posture, imagine that you, too, are painting the sky with the shining stars of your spirit. You are gracing the planet with your joyful bliss and radiating your connection to the cosmos and all that is. Say or sing out loud, *I am eternal, I am free, I'm filled with bliss and harmony.*"

Colours   Purple symbolises magic, mystery, dignity
                     and expanding imagination. It is excellent
                     for relieving headaches, promoting faith
                     and fusing Self with higher spiritual
                     awareness.

Essential Oils   A euphoric state of enlightenment can be
                     achieved via the combination of pepper-
                     mint, clove leaf and cinnamon bark. Blend
                     with sweet orange to keep you relaxed in
                     this heightened state.

Gemstones   Purple gemstones are used for meditation
                     for their cleansing and mystical
                     properties. Amethyst enhances higher
                     consciousness and repels negativity;
                     Green Agate aids decision-making; and
                     Chalcedony promotes goodwill and
                     telepathic abilities.

Sound   Choir, gospel and chill-out grooves –
                     whatever music form inspires you to look
                     to the heavens, wave your arms in the air,
                     and abandon your entire self to the feeling
                     of ecstasy. Play crystal bowls in the tone of
                     B and chant the sacred vowel of OM.

Affirmations Peace

I choose joy
Connection to bliss is easy
Miracles are all around me
Success comes easily to me
I have all the time in the world
I am a gifted child of the Universe
Ecstasy and joy are my keyword today
I am eternal, I am free,
I'm filled with bliss and harmony

Part 2:

Getting Steady

When I originally came up with this Goddess DIET, my
plan was to lose my self-loathing, gain more energy and
find peace within. Ultimately, I was successful – I
conquered my inner critic, gained my life back and
established a firm connection with my inner goddess.

What is *your* plan?

If you don't know where you want to finish up, then any
road will get you there. Let's avoid aimless meanderings
and detours and cut to the chase – to be successful with
The Goddess DIET have at least an idea of where you'd
like to finish up. Whether it's losing baggage or losing
attachment to 'ugliness', gaining self-confidence or
gaining a life, or feeling like a goddess in pajamas or a
bikini, write down your intentions before you begin.

Here are some questions you might use to start the
brainstorming:

- How I want my life to look after The Goddess DIET…

- What I need to release to align myself with this goal…
  - ☐ fear of judgement   ☐ shame
  - ☐ self-loathing   ☐ guilt
  - ☐ my inner critic   ☐ lack of self-worth
  - ☐ state of denial   ☐ Other(s)
  - ☐ subservience

- What I'm inviting in to align myself with this goal…
  - ☐ trust in self   ☐ pride
  - ☐ great intuition   ☐ joy
  - ☐ self-acceptance   ☐ self-esteem
  - ☐ total honesty   ☐ limitless energy
  - ☐ empowerment   ☐ Other(s)

Recording Your Journey

A good journal invites you to write, create, invent, explore, get lost, be found, fly, dance, spin, whisper, sing, doodle, draw, let go, find your spark and come home to your true essence. It is at once functional in that it helps you keep track of your progress, and at the same time it is a channelling tool for your divine creativity.

For The Goddess DIET, you can use your own journal or I offer you *The Goddess DIET Companion*, a handbag-sized diary tailored to receive your experiences and prompt your musings throughout your 21-day adventure. Do avoid using a journal that has sat on your bookshelf for five years because "It's too pretty to write in." (Yes, I've heard that excuse before. I've even used it once or twice myself!) Your creativity is divinely inspired and will flow whether you're using a pretty journal, a pre-formatted workbook or the back of a shopping list.

Keep a journal in your bag or near you at all times, and jot down any thoughts or messages that come to you during the next three weeks. These can be images, bullet points, mind maps or whatever 'language' makes sense to you. Don't block anything – write down everything. It doesn't even have to make sense! You'll get clarification about how you're feeling about yourself or a situation, random words or sentences that mean everything or nothing (and that's something!), images or scenes... don't discriminate, and don't be intimated by the blank page.

If you do hesitate when it comes to writing in the first page, I suggest two things: a) start on page two, and/or b) draw a squiggle. A blank page can be scary, but once the first line or doodle has been drawn, it magically absorbs that trepidation you might have about your work not being perfect or magical. Once you have started, **it is**

easy to see that yes, your creation is indeed perfect and magical, and that you too are indeed perfectly magical.

Writing in your journal does not need to be a chore. Your writing doesn't have to happen according to a prescribed style. It doesn't even need to be writing! But please, approach your journal-keeping task with tenacity and intention and the attitude will spill over to your new lifestyle explorations too. You will become better attuned to your new goddess mindset that this DIET is helping you achieve.

To succeed in this DIET, use your journal to find clues as to whether you're living authentically. Highlight synergies or contradictions between your inner world (your thoughts, feelings, emotions, values, needs and passions) and your outer world (your job, home life, circle of friends, commitments and how you spend your leisure time)? If you're not living authentically, look for clues in your writing in the form of griping, wishful thinking, impossible dreams or cynical tones. These clues point to incongruence between the way you *want* to live and the way you *actually are*. You then have a starting point for finding where you need to make changes in your life in order to achieve greater authenticity.

Make changes to what you do, how you enact your values, and how you react to situations (such as peer group pressure or expectations) that would normally have controlled your decision making processes. In doing so, you automatically gain greater personal power. Claiming your personal power means choosing to be your own super-heroine. I also call this empowered space being connected with your authentic self, tigress mother, or inner goddess. You might also resonate with words like warrior queen, earth mother, light worker, higher self or bodylicious babe. If it's right for you, it's right, period.

Elements to Record

Having said that your journal is *your* personal concern, I will venture to recommend that there are some key elements that you should include to increase the effectiveness and practicality of The Goddess DIET.

1. Benchmarks

Listen up. No matter how fat you think you are, in five years time you'll look back at photos of yourself and think, "What a whippet!" But when you look at those photos, are you able to reel off your waist size or what was going through your head at that time? Apart from "Where's my next Cosmopolitan coming from?" or "How can I lose five kilos in the next five minutes?"

In order to know how far you're getting, it helps to know where you're starting from. So on Day One of your DIET, jot down your starting measurements and weight (if that matters), or other details such as your BMI, specific baggage you want to lose, curves you want to gain, ideal states you'd like to manifest, your salary right now, items of clothing you want to fit into again, things you love or hate about yourself, the state of your health, hair, heart or hip pocket... This way, as you get further into The DIET you can track your success by revisiting your benchmarks and comparing your 'then' with your 'now'.

Even though my 'before' pic makes me cringe, it's part of my process and I'm grateful for it. As a benchmark it screams how tired, frustrated, sad and lethargic I was. Whenever I look at that photo now, instead of hating myself I am able to go to a place of gratitude. I am grateful for my restored health, I feel so wonderfully happy and blessed, and I'm delighted with how my life has turned around 180° since starting The DIET.

Anita's Benchmarks

I am currently working from 7am–2pm as a casual producer for ABC Radio. I then work from 2.15pm on my writing and my own business. Sadly, I have a power nap at about 3.30 each day – not because I want to but because my brain shuts down. I have no power over it. I am absolutely unable to rally myself out of the fog. My muscles can barely move enough to get me to the bed!

When I wake, I get back to work on my writing. Usually by 7pm I get an 11-year-old hovering behind me asking, "What's for dinner?" I then throw something together that resembles a meal and we sit and eat it together as a family – Gavstar, Boy Wonderful and me. Blaze the dyslexic god sits patiently waiting for the tell-tale sounds of scraping plates before he dares to ask for his dinner.

Gavstar does the dishes while I go back to my writing (if I'm lucky), or we sit in front of the box with a bottle of wine for a few hours, until it's time to drag ourselves to bed.

I am grumpy, stressed and feeling guilty that I can't help Gavstar more on his business. I live under a cloud that time is running out – that I have 100 books inside me that need to be written but that I will die first. I have a distrust of doctors. One wants to send me to counselling saying my exhaustion is in my head. Another wants to put me on anti-depressants.

My libido is shot, I've lost interest in socialising and waking up with sinus is the norm. This life and lifestyle is not sustainable. Despite having achieved my goals to live in a beach house and work in a career I love, I am not living my dream – deep down I am uncomfortable in my skin and have remnants of self-loathing that surface when I look in the mirror. I am at crunch time. It's time to change my choices to change my life.

2. Your Vision

Success comes easily when you can record your vision in your journal. The vision I wrote in my own journal was messy, scattered and disjointed, but it didn't matter – it only mattered that I wrote down a vision to start with. Looking back on it now, I can see that I have achieved everything my inner knowing revealed to me during a visualisation exercise.

There is a beautiful guided visualisation in my book *The Goddess Guide To Chakra Vitality (3rd edition)*, which many women use to help them access deep feelings and knowledge within. If you are so guided, use this visualisation to connect you with these answers and visions with which to create your own vision. It is also available as an mp3 download via TheGoddessDiet.com if you would prefer to listen to the visualisation rather than read it.

Read your preferred guided visualisation in a quiet space, with gentle music in the background, and with your intention attuned to your success. Alternatively, have a friend read it to you while you close your eyes and visualise your journey along the path to enlightenment. Yet another idea is to record the visualisation onto your mp3 player and listen to it at your leisure, in your easy chair, with your phone switched off and a refreshing glass of water by your side.

During most visualisations you will be prompted to acknowledge, verbalise, describe or recognise answers that lie dormant within you, thereby bypassing sub-conscious blockages or habits of self-sabotage.

Whenever an answer pops into your head, do not second-guess it, wonder where it came from or shut it down... simply remember it so that you can write it down in your journal once you've completed the visualisation. It might not make sense right now, but it doesn't have to. Be open to the messages that will be presenting themselves to you during this process – they all have their place in unlocking and unleashing the miraculous You within.

At your own pace, record your messages, visions, feelings and emotions into your journal. You may only have one word, one image, or an entire story… everyone is different. Take all the time in your world to do this, and do not disconnect from your journey until you feel at peace with what you have set free.

You'Here are some prompts for when it comes to putting your vision into words:

- I see myself…
- I feel that I am…
- When I (do this), I (react this way)…
- I know I am successful because…
- My secret weapon is…
- I am surrounded by…
- It is easy to…
- As a warrior queen I…
- My purpose is to…
- My personal motto is…

Pssst. If you're too busy for this, then you're too busy to take charge of your new life as a fully-fledged, self-actualised goddess. If your excuse is that you can't meditate, try reading my book *Sacred Vigilance, Wide-Awake Meditation.* Any more excuses? Goddess sister, I don't mean to sounds harsh, but please only embark on this journey when you are *ready* to shine. That means aligning your intention to that of success. ☺

Anita's Vision

I see myself glowing with health. I see myself fitting comfortably in my clothes. I feel my waist and it is in the shape of an hourglass, sturdy and strong. I see the muscles in my legs coping easily with hikes. My ankles have shape! I feel the air in my lungs revive me naturally. My hair behaves each morning. No-one bumps into me at market-places and I don't have to jostle for service at cafés. I am actually visible!

I see myself sitting on a front step in the sunshine. People say hello as they walk past. I feel like an essential being in the matrix of humanity. I am taller than ever before. I am more graceful than ever before. I see smiles on strangers when I pass them in the street. I see glimpses of my inner spectacular wow factor and can access that power at any time. I see people asking for my advice. I sense when they are hiding something, even from themselves. I know exactly when to say yes. My words are valued. Mother Nature talks directly to me, and I see her infinite beauty in every cloud, pebble and pine needle. Chocolate is good for me. I also see myself enjoying fruit. I am grateful for the abundance of good food waiting for me to enjoy it. I know that the farmers who produced it do so because of their love for the land, Mother Nature and me. I see them intuitively connected with the earth's cycles and feel energised by the same connection. "Yes" is my favourite word and it serves me perfectly. I see myself enjoying only a small glass of boutique wine each day, and lots of locally-grown produce. Water is everywhere – in the rivers we cross, the creeks I jump, the oceans we paddle in and in the snow on the mountain tops. I know that water is instantly reviving and I see myself drinking it regularly.

I see myself smiling. My son is a reflection of my perfection. My man is proud to share my joy. The three of us smile together. It is easy to smile because I am deeply, profoundly, genuinely and soul-quenchingly happy.

3. Your Pledge to Self

The next step in preparing yourself for The Goddess DIET is to identify key aspects of messages obtained during your visualisation and use them to formulate a pledge to your Self. Allow unconditional love to flow through you as you prioritise your needs.

What are you going to absolutely and positively promise yourself at a heart felt level? Is physical comfort a key reward you'd like to gift yourself? Perhaps you have residual guilt or pain you'd like to heal. Or maybe you just want to have more fun and spontaneity in your life.

Written words contain innate power – they cement your intentions and make them real. Whatever your desire, take the first step in achieving it by creating and writing a stunning, easy pledge to your Self. For example, I wrote my pledge in third person to my inner child and inner goddess. It was:

To my dear Anita,

You deserve to feel unrestricted in your clothes, enjoy unlimited energy, and to appreciate your glorious Self in all your aspects.

In my choices and actions over the next 21 days I fully intend to gift these successes to you.

With all my love and oodles more,
your tigress mother.
xx

In writing down this promise I immediately felt obliged to succeed – not because cheating would make me a liar, but because in formalising my promise I realised that the outcome of this pledge was something I really, really, *really* wanted to give myself.

Referring back to the pledge during times of temptation helped steel my resolve during times I would otherwise have cheated on The DIET… let's face it, there are some days a cream bun or a glass of stars is the answer to your prayers.

Your pledge will become a valuable resource. Think of it as your Goddess Creed[41] – a short statement that sums up your intention and ideals. For example, my creed during The Goddess DIET became:

> *I am fit, fluid and fabulous,*
> *open, aware and wise*

In another example of what a pledge can look like, in *The 7-Day Chakra Workout* I suggest writing a pledge in first person to own the promise on a personal level. It is:

> *In seeking to accomplish a positive life, I hereby*
> *align my intention with the vision of that*
> *which I seek to attract.*

Increase your resolution and your intention by formulating your pledge-to-Self in your journal.

You can explore the following propositions if you need further prompting, but I suggest you return again and again to the messages you received during your visualisation in order to tune into your intuitive direction.

4. The Four Rs

And now for the daily nitty gritty: keeping track of four essential aspects of a healthy life: **Real Food, Recreation, Rest and Reflection**. I absolutely recommend that you journal these aspects each day to ensure you keep it all in balance – great food, enjoyable exercise, heavenly repose and a heightened intention to have a fabulous life.

Real Food

Janine Allis, CEO of Boost Juice[42], says that choosing real food is "as simple as dividing food into two food groups – processed and unprocessed, or natural and unnatural." Keep this is mind as you're choosing your food during the 21 days while you're on The Goddess DIET.

Furthermore, if you've forgotten the essential principles of choosing healthy meals, revisit Tool 14: Burnout Buster in the Body of Evidence section of this book.

And finally, there is one other method you can use when making healthy food choices: *use your intuition*.

After dozens of visits to three different doctors and dozens of blood tests to find out why I was soooo tired all the time, deep down I suspected my weight-gain-energy-loss problem was food-related. Or more to the point, an intolerance to a food group.

To confirm what my intuition was telling me, I visited a kinesiologist. Kinesiology is a form of natural health care which combines the principles of Chinese medicine with muscle monitoring to assess energy and body function.

Before I embarked on my 21-day vacation, I enlisted the help of my aunty (a kinesiologist) on Christmas Day, in between the three course breakfast and the six-course lunch. I valued her opinion and wanted her thoughts on:

- why I was feeling so lousy;
- how I could fix my daily hay fever symptoms;
- how to relieve the persistent heaviness in my gut;
- ways to increase my energy and clarity; and
- which foods might be culprit and which foods were my 'friends'.

The results were pretty close to what I'd already intuited for myself – I had developed an intolerance to gluten and to a lesser extent, dairy products.

I let our findings be my guide when reading menus rather than succumbing to my (sometimes) naughty taste buds. Over the 21 days I found that more and more, my intuition and taste buds gradually became more congruent with each other, and choosing the right foods for my body subsequently became easier and easier.

Recreation

Packing your bags and heading to new territory is a wonderful reason to strap on your hiking shoes – you have thousands of fresh streets to explore, different shops to browse and new horizons to appreciate. Taking the new scenery in your stride will mean you're exercising without even realising.

If you can't leave town, make a daily visit to the gym, park, pool or pilates class your break-from-routine.

Even if your intention during your break-from-routine is to laze by a pool reading a book, at least this is helping you relax and revitalise. It's also feeding valuable sunlight to your body, which produces serotonin – a feel-good hormone that lessens your cravings for sugar and junk food. Just make sure that at the very least you *swim* to the bar, or you do a few extra laps of the pool (either in it or around the edge) to get your metabolism one notch above frozen. And remember, 100 ankle twirls or calf stretches may not make up for the six Cosmopolitans that you sip throughout the day, but if you lose weight while singing karaoke wrapped in plastic let me know!

Rest

While your current life may be crazy and mad busy, the beauty of going on vacation is that you can take at least an hour a day on your holidays to sit and 'be' with your surroundings. I can't reiterate enough how important it is to grab 30 minutes of Goddess Time every day. Without it, you remain a slave to your routine, to others' demands and in the loop of stress. Stress causes our adrenal glands to release a hormone called cortisol.

Cortisol "…makes us store fat in case of famine," says David Cameron-Smith, Associate Professor in Nutrition Sciences at Deakin University in Melbourne[43].

So, stress = cortisol = fat storage. Not only that, it gives us a jelly belly – the fat gain tends to become concentrated around the abdomen. The solution is to increase your exercise, recreation and 'me time' to spark the release of beta-endorphins – brain chemicals which improve mood and promote calm. As such, Goddess Time prevents jelly belly. It helps alleviate the stress on your adrenal glands and enables you to come back to a balanced and more peaceful space.

Now, there's another aspect of Rest that is as important as Goddess Time, and that is: **sleep**. Sleep deprivation can increase the hormone that stimulates appetite (ghrelin), and decrease the hormone that makes us feel full (leptin). So get lots of zeds to help produce more leptin – not only does it suppress your appetite, but the rest recharges your batteries and rouses you to get active.

Scientific stuff aside, a nap is wonderful for charging your batteries. Winston Churchill is a famous napper who got through the stresses of World War II with a nap each afternoon. He is in the company of Thomas Edison who took nano-naps (naps that last less than two minutes) to daydream new solutions to old problems.

Naps open your consciousness to revelations not visible on the physical plane. It is when you are in the halfway world between lucidity and sleep that the subliminal workings of your mind presents you with fresh ideas and previously unthought-of insights. Harness this energy to gain new perspectives on old ruts.

Reflection

Reflecting on Self, directions and values helps bring clarity and a greater sense of purpose to our lives. Insights gained by being conscious and present are gifts to bring more meaning to the way we live.

Each day during the 21 days, read the short reflection provided in Part 3 of this book. A summary of these reflections is on the next page.

See these reflections as launching pads for revealing new depths to your emotions, creativity and inner wisdom.

Use your journal to record your thoughts and reactions to the key aspect of that reflection. For example, when you read reflections designed to inspire your warrior queen, reflect on ways this archetype connects you with the life aspect of security. What is lacking in your that you don't feel settled? What do you have in abundance that does make you feel safe? How can you feel a stronger connection to your family and neighbours? And so on.

Reflections For Each Goddess Archetype

These meditations are based on the essential life aspects facing every woman. In all cases, ask yourself, "What would the archetypal goddess do in this situation?" and journal your thoughts, feelings and reactions.

The reflections I worked with during my own journey (in no particular order) are as follows:

Archetype	Key Life Aspects
Warrior Queen	• Passion / Apathy • Security / Lack of Direction • Community / Disconnection
Magical Muse	• Change / Inertia • Nourishment / Abuse • Laughter / Melancholy
Daring Diva	• Boundaries / Exploitation • Individuality / Monochrome • Personal Power / Manipulation
Primordial Mother	• Love / Fear • Light / Regret • Generosity / Greed
Natural Healer	• Honesty / Denial • Integrity / Pretence • Assertion / Repression
Sacred Sage	• Reinvention / Boredom • Certainty / Procrastination • Consciousness / Indifference
High Priestess	• Bliss / Gloom • Gratitude / Blame • Wisdom / Ignorance

Part 3:

Let the

Transformation Begin!

Day 1 :: Warrior Queen

Mood

Body Tools

Mind Tools

Spirit Tools

Affirmation   *I am surrounded by friends and family*
                  who support me unconditionally.

What I Saw
in the Mirror

Real Food

Rest

Recreation

Reflection: The first community we know is our family.
Community As we grow up we enter a play group, then
school, then sporting teams and after-
school activities. We launch into adulthood
and gravitate to social, work or more global
communities – groups of like-minded
people with aligned passions and ideals.
Even online, thousands of communities
foster relationships that validate our
thoughts and ethics. Being part of a
community is a primal urge instilled from
birth. Meet your neighbours, smile at
people in your street, get involved in local
events, share your resources, ask for help,
recognise loneliness in others and work to
alleviate it.

Answer this question in your journal: What
would a warrior queen do to foster her
community?

Day 2 :: Magical Muse

Mood

Body Tools

Mind Tools

Spirit Tools

Affirmation   *My body is sacred,*
                   a treasure and a pleasure

**What I Saw
in the Mirror**

Real Food

Rest

Recreation

Reflection: The funny thing about the body is, unless it
Self-Care   complains we tend to take it for granted.
               But in taking it for granted we give it cause
               to complain!

               The body is our vehicle for life, and just like
               a car it is important to keep it tuned. Its
               needs are quite simple, readily available
               and a lot cheaper than petrol: good food,
               water, enjoyable exercise and rest. See these
               four elements as nourishment for your
               body rather than tools to fulfil an emotional
               hunger or void. Balance your food and
               fitness, recreation and rest, and your body
               will be good for miles and miles and
               miles...

               Answer this question in your journal: What
               are a magical muse's favourite ways to
               nourish herself?

Day 3 :: Daring Diva

Mood

Body Tools

Mind Tools

Spirit Tools

Affirmation *My boundaries are clear*
so I have nothing to fear

**What I Saw
in the Mirror**

Real Food

Rest

Recreation

Reflection: Sometimes we find ourselves modifying
Boundaries our behaviour to suit others. Some
compromise is fine, but if you're denying
your needs to avoid rejection or to keep the
peace, you are sending the message that
your needs aren't worthy of fulfilment.
Setting boundaries shows others how they
can or cannot treat you and gives them
permission to treat you with the respect
you deserve. In order to make boundaries
effective, decide on suitable consequences
in response to exploitive behaviour. A
consequence is not a punishment or a threat
but a statement of what you will do if such
behaviour continues. Be prepared to carry
out the consequence in order to restore your
personal power.

Answer this question in your journal: How
does a daring diva establish boundaries?

Day 4 :: Primordial Mother

Mood

Body Tools

Mind Tools

Spirit Tools

Affirmation   *In benevolence I believe;*
so that in giving I receive
for the greatest good all.

**What I Saw
in the Mirror**

Real Food

Rest

Recreation

Reflection: The Universal law of three-fold means the
Generosity more you give away, the more that comes
back to you. Sounds good in theory, but
there is a catch… you can't give something
away with the motivation that it's scoring
you karmic points.

When you give your time, energy or
material items, release any ulterior motives
for personal gain; make sure your gift is
from a place of true benevolence. After all,
generosity is about sharing your resources
for the greatest good of all. To think
otherwise is a self-centred act rooted in
greed, and is bound to backfire.

Answer this question in your journal: What
can a primordial mother do to demonstrate
selfless generosity?

Day 5 :: Natural Healer

Mood

_____

Body Tools

_____

Mind Tools

_____

Spirit Tools

_____

Affirmation   *I am able to say what I think,*
                  and do what I say.

_____

What I Saw
in the Mirror

_____

Real Food

Rest

Recreation

Reflection:
Integrity

Socrates taught "The greatest way to live with honour ... is to be what we pretend to be." His lesson promotes the quality of integrity – actually be-ing the good person we appear to be, and do-ing what is right rather than what is convenient. Any departure from integrity means you're just pretending. Pretence attracts pretence in equal measure; your reward for insincerity is superficial relationships, artificial luck and a sham reality. Integrity is when what you think, say and do all align. You can fulfil promises because you have the mettle to carry out good intentions. You are reliable because of your consistent adherence to being real. And you are trustworthy because you live your truth.

Answer this question in your journal: How does a natural healer act with integrity?

Day 6 :: Sacred Sage

Mood

Body Tools

Mind Tools

Spirit Tools

Affirmation   *I care.*

**What I Saw
in the Mirror**

Real Food

Rest

Recreation

Reflection: Are you living your life in ignorance or
Awareness   indifference? (Don't let your answer be "I
              don't know and I don't care," ha ha.)

              Dare to care about your life choices and
              direction. Pay attention about where you're
              heading, what you're doing and who
              you're sharing your Self with. Be conscious
              of the many small miracles that happen
              around you every day. Take notice of
              synchronicities. Enter portals in time. See
              the symbolism in numbers, visions and
              happenchance. Increase your awareness of
              your essence and how it melds or offsets
              with others. All of these things hold clues to
              your spiritual well-being.

              Answer this question in your journal: How
              does a sacred sage behave when she is
              behaving consciously?

Day 7 :: High Priestess

Mood

Body Tools

Mind Tools

Spirit Tools

Affirmation *Thank you*

**What I Saw
in the Mirror**

Real Food

Rest

Recreation

Reflection: Be thankful for the little blessings that
Gratitude   present themselves to you hundreds of
times a day. When your attention is on
being grateful for a warm bed, hot food,
laughing children and even running water,
you are charging your Self with positive
power. Taking notice of the thousands of
gifts on offer each day becomes your focus
and takes priority over hardships, hurts
and blame. Blaming others for their
transgressions, your material lack or
problems in general only serves to keep
that situation in focus. Hardships make us
stronger so change your attitude to that of
gratitude and you'll soon be showering in
blessings and good fortune.

Answer this question in your journal: How
many blissings can a high priestess handle
in one day? List them all!

Day 8 :: Warrior Queen

Mood

Body Tools

Mind Tools

Spirit Tools

Affirmation   *I am passionate about the right projects*
                  for the right reasons

What I Saw
in the Mirror

Real Food

Rest

Recreation

Reflection: Every great venture has been fuelled by
Passion passion. A project can't come to fruition
without your enthusiasm and willingness
to act on your vision – this is your passion
in action. Passion is 'working' to ensure the
future of your life, a person or a project, but
it's a fun and satisfying pursuit. Having
passion means you are able to become
emotional about your existence and you
can revisit the carefree enthusiasm for life
you enjoyed as a child. 'Work' becomes
play, and play is joyous and easy. If you're
feeling apathetic about a project or a
situation, it's time to either let it go or find a
new angle that will stir your passion for its
success.

Answer this question in your journal: When
you are warrior queen personified, what is
your greatest passion?

Day 9 :: Magical Muse

Mood

Body Tools

Mind Tools

Spirit Tools

Affirmation *Giggle and chuckle, chortle and shout,*
laughing helps me let it all out!

**What I Saw
in the Mirror**

Real Food

Rest

Recreation

Reflection: No matter what your culture, laughter is
Laughter the Universal language of joy. It is your
body's way of releasing anxiety, fear and
stress to replace them with feel-good
hormones and eustress (the 'good' stress).
Life's problems become trivial in the light
of a good laugh. Suddenly it is easy to look
on the bright side of sad situations and
melancholy becomes just a passing phase.
Actively seek external triggers to help you
laugh – see a comedy at the movies, share a
giggle with a friend, read the comic strips,
watch children at play. If all else fails, fake
it. Chuckle, chortle, giggle, snort or guffaw,
and the infectious nature of laughter will
take over soon enough.

Answer this question in your journal: Oh
beautiful and succulent muse, where are
you going to get a laugh from today?

Day 10 :: Daring Diva

Mood

Body Tools

Mind Tools

Spirit Tools

Affirmation   *Power up oh magnificent me!*

**What I Saw
in the Mirror**

Real Food

Rest

Recreation

Reflection:
Identity
It is traditional for us to wish on the first star we see each evening, but isn't it wonderful to gaze upon the cascade of stars that follow? Each and every star is as unique and magnificent to look upon as its neighbour, yet part of the beauty of individuality is being able to delight in the diversity of others also. Each star plays its own role as part of the 'big picture' whilst maintaining its own integral position in the Universe. You can do the same in your own life. Allow yourself to be the splash of colour that brightens a monochrome landscape. See faces in the crowd. Wear a flower in your hair. Relish your quirks. In short, be yourself – there's no-one better qualified.

Answer this question in your journal: Daring and darling diva, who are you?

Day 11 :: Primordial Mother

Mood

_____

Body Tools

_____

Mind Tools

_____

Spirit Tools

_____

Affirmation   *I am light, bright and outta sight!*

_____

What I Saw
in the Mirror

_____

Real Food

Rest

Recreation

Reflection:
Light

'Light' is a desirable state of being in our vernacular. To feel as 'light as air' is to be able to drift with the winds of fortune without encumbrance or remorse; to 'light up the stage' is to gift others with our radiant, luminous presence; and to 'travel light' is to be able to journey through life without emotional baggage and regrets. Regrets about missed opportunities or 'bad' behaviour may weigh us down but do deserve recognition for the lessons they hold. Acknowledge regrets, then let them pass with gratitude for the lesson. Invite lightness into your life: unclutter your physical and emotional world, clear out negative words and energy and welcome in things and thoughts that make you glow.

Answer this question in your journal: As a primordial mother, what makes you glow?

Day 12 :: Natural Healer

Mood

Body Tools

Mind Tools

Spirit Tools

Affirmation   *My needs are heard and met*

**What I Saw
in the Mirror**

Real Food

Rest

Recreation

Reflection: No-one likes conflict, yet we face some
Assertion   form of it every day. Whether it's internal or
              going on around us, sometimes it's just
              easier to 'put up and shut up' than to share
              how we really feel about a situation.

              News flash: ignoring the situation does not
              make it go away. Speaking up might feel
              like the scarier option in resolving conflict,
              but it is certainly the healthiest option for
              achieving peace of mind. Channel
              repressed feelings into creating positive,
              affirmative statements about how the
              situation is affecting you, and how you'd
              like to see it resolved. Assert your need for
              respect in the situation with calm and
              measured energy in order to be heard.

              Answer this question in your journal: How
              are you going to be heard today?

Day 13 :: Sacred Sage

Mood

_____

Body Tools

_____

Mind Tools

_____

Spirit Tools

_____

Affirmation *Just do it!*

_____

**What I Saw
in the Mirror**

_____

Real Food

Rest

Recreation

Reflection: We're all faced with impossible decisions at
Certainty   times, or it may just be that procrastination
is blocking your progress. Don't put off
until tomorrow what could have been done
yesterday. If you'd just done it when you
were supposed to, your 'inbox' would be
clear today! Be certain about what it is you
want to achieve, which direction you'd like
to take, and how you want each outcome to
enrich your life. Do not get distracted with
chit-chat or web surfing. Do not wander off
and begin other tasks. Visualise yourself
completing your task at hand, then do it!
Trust that each decision you make from
intuition will result in your highest good,
and then get on with the job!

Answer this question in your journal: Now
that you are thinking clearly, what jobs are
you going to clear from your to-do list?

Day 14 :: High Priestess

Mood

Body Tools

Mind Tools

Spirit Tools

Affirmation   *My eyes are open as is my heart,*
I am always ready for the learning to start

**What I Saw
in the Mirror**

Real Food

Rest

Recreation

Reflection: *Wisdom*	There are many kinds of knowledge: cognitive, intuitive, intellectual, spiritual, creative and emotional. Each form is energised differently – business acumen is ruled by the left-brain, for example, whereas spiritual and creative wisdom belongs more to the right-brain realm. You were born with your own style of innate wisdom which continues to grow every day. Whether your knowledge comes from listening to others, reading books, watching how it's done, or rolling up your sleeves and doing it by trial and error, strive to remain open to learning something new every day to avoid becoming stale and ignorant.
	Answer this question in your journal: Wise and wonderful high priestess, what have you learned and shared today?

Day 15 :: Warrior Queen

Mood

Body Tools

Mind Tools

Spirit Tools

Affirmation *My path reveals itself to me*
at the perfect time
in the perfect way

**What I Saw
in the Mirror**

Real Food

Rest

Recreation

Reflection:
Security

Being grounded and secure is the one of the fundamental principles in Maslow's hierarchy of needs, (second to the needs to breathe, dispose of bodily wastes, regulate body temperature and get adequate food, water and sleep. Your sense of security comes under threat when events beyond your control send you into a spiral: death, divorce, a child leaving home, a major illness, loss of a job or a best friend...

See this state of chaos as an opportunity to release attachments to how you think things 'should be', and to accept that exciting possibilities are preparing to shower them-selves upon you.

Answer this question in your journal: What makes a warrior queen feel safe and secure?

Day 16 :: Magical Muse

Mood

Body Tools

Mind Tools

Spirit Tools

Affirmation *Onwards and upwards!*

**What I Saw
in the Mirror**

Real Food

Rest

Recreation

Reflection:
Change

Change is inevitable (except from a vending machine). Everything around you and within you changes – it evolves, progresses, regresses and morphs. It is only when we resist change that it becomes a problem. It's natural to want to stand your ground and wrap yourself in all that is familiar, but remember, the only reason to be afraid of change is if you think things are going to get worse. Change your mind about change. It brings with it new opportunities, creative energy and a fresh outlook. Open the curtains on your musty life, shed some light on old issues that keep you stuck in your rut and step outside your comfort zone to see how things can only get better.

Answer this question in your journal: How is the magical muse going to challenge her comfort zone today?

Day 17 :: Daring Diva

Mood

Body Tools

Mind Tools

Spirit Tools

Affirmation *I am my own personal heroine*

What I Saw in the Mirror

Real Food

Rest

Recreation

Reflection: Confidence is maintaining an expectation
Personal for a positive outcome. Allowing negative
Power thoughts, people or experiences to creep in
undermines your right to happiness. When
you feel butterflies in your gut, this is your
fight or flight mechanism kicking in to
protect you from those trying to manipulate
you. They may be using bullying tactics, or
deflecting their fears or guilt onto you so
that you will behave a certain way. See
yourself as a mirror and deflect these
negative energies away from you. Be
persistent in your goal for empowerment
and reclaim your right to make your own
choices, to be your own Self, and to expect
the best.

Answer this question in your journal: What
are the butterflies in your belly really telling
you, and what will the diva do about it?

Day 18 :: Primordial Mother

Mood

Body Tools

Mind Tools

Spirit Tools

Affirmation   *I step into love, love, love*

**What I Saw
in the Mirror**

Real Food

Rest

Recreation

Reflection: *Love*	There are only two forces in the Universe that influence your decision-making and values: love and fear.

You have the choice to act from either space. Hold the scales of justice in your hand and place what can be *gained* with love on one side (the three G-forces of Love: Gratitude, Grace and Generosity), and what can be *lost* with love on the other side, (the Three Heartbreak-Rs: Regrets, Reproach and Retribution). See how love is all-powerful? If your scales ever tip towards fear, consciously step into a space of love. Know you are supported by the Universe's greatest power.

Explore this prompt in your journal: What situation can be changed by acting from a space of mother love rather than fear?

Day 19 :: *Natural Healer*

Mood

Body Tools

Mind Tools

Spirit Tools

Affirmation   *I know truth, I speak truth, I am truth*

**What I Saw
in the Mirror**

Real Food

Rest

Recreation

Reflection: "Above all else to thine own self be true,"
Honesty says Shakespeare. In your heart of hearts, you know when you are lying to yourself and so does your sub-conscious and soul. Go to the heart of the matter whenever you feel doubt or fear. What is the limiting belief that is preventing you from succeeding? Use your intuition to listen to your body and have the courage to act on it. The Goddess DIET requires that you pull off your Mask-of-Denial and be absolutely above board and honest with yourself. Even if you fudge the scales or sneak a sinful snack, you can't get away with being dishonest with yourself. Speak your truth, act your truth, be your truth.

Answer this question in your journal: What is the natural healer going to admit to herself today?

Day 20 :: Sacred Sage

Mood

Body Tools

Mind Tools

Spirit Tools

Affirmation   *I have the resources I need*
                  when I need them

**What I Saw
in the Mirror**

Real Food

Rest

Recreation

Reflection:
Reinvention

Every day we are required to be different people in order to cope with different demands – sometimes we need to be a tigress mother to defend our little ones, at other times we become a butterfly at social events, and on Sunday mornings we can be a sloth lazing until late morning. It is perfectly natural to marshal energy from different inspiration sources to bring excitement and new gifts to each situation. Transcend the pitfalls of stagnancy (boredom, decay, self-loathing) by refreshing your outlook, renewing your goals and reinventing your Self. Aim to embody the qualities you can appreciate to the utmost.

Answer this question in your journal: How is the sacred sage going to reinvent herself today?

Day 21 :: High Priestess

Mood

Body Tools

Mind Tools

Spirit Tools

Affirmation *Regardless of what my future holds,*
I embrace each day as it unfolds,
I am thankful for the sun's sweet kiss,
And all the things that bring me bliss

**What I Saw
in the Mirror**

Real Food

Rest

Recreation

Reflection: The chrysanthemum is a plant that
Bliss   flourishes more freely if it is pinched back
                 in the springtime – this is the process
                 whereby the growing shoots are slightly
                 damaged in order to promote more
                 vigourous growth outwards. It is an
                 interesting analogy to our own lives.
                 Providing you see each obstacle as a lesson
                 rather than a hindrance, you can grow
                 naturally stronger with each adversity you
                 overcome. It is completely OK to hibernate
                 in a cave while you rejuvenate, but follow
                 this period of introspection with lots of
                 healing laughter to surmount the gloom
                 and achieve a state of bliss.

                 Answer this question in your journal: Oh
                 beautiful and wise high priestess, you have
                 nourished your body, mind and soul for 21
                 days. How are you going to celebrate?

Resources and Yummy-ohs

The Goddess DIET Companion

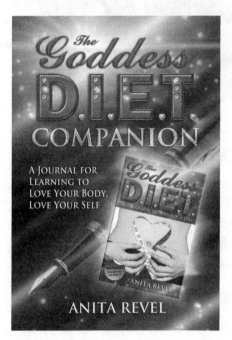

This is a journal and workbook to help you love your body, love your Self. It is the perfect companion in which to record your musings as you journey through The Goddess DIET. Write, create, invent, explore, get lost, be found, fly, dance, spin, whisper, sing, doodle, draw, let go, find your spark and come home to your true essence.

The Chakra Goddess Visualisation

Anita Revel's guided visualisation through the chakras features in her book, *The Goddess Guide to Chakra Vitality*, and also in Goddess Playshops – workshops for women's well-being. Listen to the visualisation to access deep feelings and knowledge within, and be open to receiving divinely channelled messages throughout this 21-minute chakra journey. The beautiful Chakra Goddess Visualisation is now available as an mp3 download from various websites including TheGoddessDiet.com

Other Books by Anita Revel

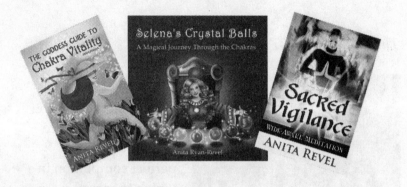

The Goddess Guide to Chakra Vitality (3rd edition)

Through honouring the feminine divine, we reconnect with our inner goddess. We respect and empower ourselves spiritually, psychologically, emotionally, and physically. Keeping our chakras energised nurtures the inner goddess and achieves balance in our lives.

Selena's Crystal Balls (illustrated book for children)

Foster your child's emotional intelligence with this illustrated journey through the colours of the rainbow. The story encourages children to check in with the energy of colours, and to establish associations between colours, emotions, imagery and the seven essential aspects of life.

Sacred Vigilance, Wide Awake Meditation

Sacred Vigilance™ is an easy meditation style that doesn't involve quiet space, rhythmic breathing, chanting, sub-consciousness, fasting, slowing, or anywhere-in-betweening. It can be done anywhere, any time – at the gym, at a café, in the supermarket queue. And perhaps best of all, it's fun to do. You only need one minute, one hour or one afternoon to manifest abundance and happiness for all, including your beautiful Self.

Journals and Workbooks by Anita Revel

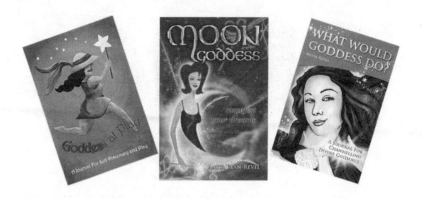

Goddess At Play, Journal For Self-Discovery and Play

This journal is your receptacle for messages and insights you receive during a Goddess Playshop™. Reconnect your Self, intuition and Spirit, and see your Self as a perfect reflection of the ancient goddess archetypes. Created exclusively for Goddess Playshops Pty Ltd.

Moon Goddess, Manifest Your Dreams

By increasing your awareness of the moon's intuitive, emotional and compelling gifts, you can deepen your connection with your own feminine wisdom and power. In this easy-to-read guide and workbook, Anita Ryan-Revel explores the many ways you can start new projects and manifest your dreams, by reconnecting with moon and goddess energies.

What Would Goddess Do?

This is a journal for channelling divine guidance. Restore balance and magic to your life by celebrating the highs and documenting the lows. Explore, create, play, ignite, animate and stimulate your divine spark with rampant gusto and grace. That's what goddess would do.

About the Author

As described on Anita's website (AnitaRevel.com), Anita is a creatrix, author, mother and wife, web diva, dream weaver, lover of life. She's also a marriage celebrant, teacher, artist, traveller and joy junkie but couldn't make these rhyme. Nevertheless, all these roles pretty well sum up her passion for inspired living.

During the early stages of her journey, Anita's appetite for new experiences saw her become a scientist, marketing director, Japanese teacher, and whatever else took her fancy. In 1996 she answered her calling to immerse herself in true, full-tilt living, and subsequently embarked on a conscious quest to honour her higher Self in all aspects of life. As such, Anita's work is aimed at helping you connect with your beautiful, sassy, intuitive, lovable, sacred and authentic Self – your inner goddess.

In 2005, Anita became the Creatrix of the internationally popular Goddess Playshop™ (which feature her gorgeous Goddess-ence 100% pure essential oil blends).

She is also the author of a growing collection of well-being resources, countless columns for United Press International, hundreds of articles found sprinkled across the internet, and numerous books.

Anita lives on a farm in the stunning Margaret River region of Western Australia with her husband and two children. Her favourite time of day is watching the sun set like a glob of golden butter into the Indian Ocean, even if it does make her hungry for popcorn.

Thanks to a very fertile 2007 and productive 2008, many more books and products are being manifested in 2009.

Gratitude and Blessings

No journey is complete without the support and inspiration from co-travellers, co-goddesses, co-operation and coffee. So here is where I thank everyone who inspired me, nagged me, begged me and pushed me to finish this four-year project and share my secrets for holistic well-being.

To my co-travellers... my husband, two children and Blaze the dyslexic god. To use a cliché (forgive me!) words aren't enough to express my gratitude for your patience and support. I might even help out with the dishes now that this project has been birthed (but no promises, you hear?).

To my co-goddesses... Natalie, Mama Gena and Sharon in the northern hemisphere, and Serene, Lucy, Maria and Trudy in the southern. Whether your words have appeared in this book or not, your ideas, feedback and wisdom have influenced me to write the way I do.

To my co-operators... the associate professors and researchers who took the time to respond to my endless queries; Janet for picking the draft to pieces; Rebecca for her patience with the dozens of cover tweaks; my goddess sisters who so kindly and generously offered testimonials; and Scott for not recognising me after my second journey (post pregnancy) through The Goddess DIET – this is the ultimate testimony to the transform-ation I underwent.

And to the bottomless cups of coffee... I hope you'll forgive me for dividing my time between you, chocolate, cheese and champagne – I didn't want to limit how much love I could cram into each day.

Love love love you lots!

Resources and Cited Sources

1 The Yale School of Medicine's research on synaptic
   connections was published in The Journal of
   Neuroscience 27: 9951-9961 (October 2007)

2 Janice Taylor is a weight-loss coach based in New York.
   OurLadyOfWeightLoss.com

3 The Daily Blissings Project can be found at
   CountYourBlissings.com

4 The Better Health Channel is a health and medical
   information service quality assured by the Victorian
   government.

5 Better Health Channel website: Betterhealth.vic.gov.au

6 According to Okinawa-Diet.com, Okinawans register
   80 percent less heart disease than United States citizens.

7 The report by the Department of Chemical Engineering
   at the Jordan University of Science and Technology was
   published at pubs.acs.org/cgi-bin/sample.cgi/iecred/
   2007/46/i16/html/ie070527l.html

8 Doctor Rodney Ford is also known as Doctor Gluten
   because of his expertise in The Gluten Syndrome.
   DoctorGluten.com

9 The report on comfort foods and the chronically stressed
   was published at Sciencedaily.com/releases/
   2003/09/030911072109.htm

10 The Slow Food Organisation is a non-profit group
    founded in Italy to counteract fast food and fast life. Join
    the revolution at SlowFood.com

11 Bruce M. Spiegelman of the Dana-Farber Cancer Institute says body fat is necessary for healthy body functions. dana-farber.org

12 Goddesstrology defines us and our life purpose. Download a free iPhone app: GoddessBirthSigns.com

13 Wahlqvist, M.L. (ed). 2002. *Food and Nutrition*, Allen and Unwin

14 Wahlqvist, M.L.(ed). 1997. *Food and Nutrition, Australasia, Asia and the Pacific.* Chapter 30: Foods, physical activity and sport.

15 The researchers at at the University of Washington School of Medicine have proven carbohydrates should not be overly restricted in any diet. uwmedicine.org

16 A research team at Indiana University recommends exercise within an hour of eating. hper.indiana.edu

17 The United States Department of Agriculture has a comprehensive online database of nutrient profiles for 13,000 foods at usda.gov ('Food and Nutrition')

18 Don Tolmans' whole food signatures can be found at dontolmaninternational.com

19 Institute of Food Technologists: ift.org

20 Great Moments in Science: abc.net.au/science/k2/moments/s341437.htm

21 A team at the Mayo Clinic in Rochester found that people who fidget put on less fat than the couch potatoes. mayoresearch.mayo.edu/mayo/research/pubsearch.cfm

22 Levine JA, et al. (1999). *Role of nonexercise activity thermogenesis in resistance to fat gain in humans.* Science, 283, 212-214.

23 Levine JA, et al. (2005). Interindividual variation in
    posture allocation: possible role in human obesity.
    Science, 307, 584-586.

24 The Australian government recommend 2.5 hours of
    moderate exercise a week. ausport.gov.au/fulltext/1999/
    feddep/physguide.pdf

25 2000 steps to weight-loss... The University of Colorado
    Health Sciences Center uchsc.edu/news/bridge/2004/
    December/weightloss.html

26 UK journalist Nicky Taylor drank 516 units of alcohol
    over 30 days and aged 11 years. bbc.co.uk/bbcthree/
    programmes/mischief/series_one/booze_bird

27 The Albert Einstein College of Medicine: aecom.yu.edu/
    home/research.asp

28 Chen, H. J., Karlsson, C. and Povey, M. J. W. (2005),
    Acoustic Envelop Detector for Crispness Assessment of
    Biscuits, J. Text. Stud. 36, 139-156

29 Author Shakti Gawain is in semi-retirement, according to
    her staff, but you can still find out more about Creative
    Visualisation via her website, shaktigawain.com

30 Maria Elita is a life coach and author based in
    Queensland, Australia. MariaElita.com

31 Norcross, J, Mrykalo, M, Blagys, M. *Auld Lang Syne:
    Success predictors, change processes, and self-reported
    outcomes of New Year's resolvers and nonresolvers,,*
    University of Scranton. Journal of Clinical Psychology,
    Volume 58, Issue 4 (2002).

32 A Goddess Playshop™ is a two-hour workshop for
    women's well-being. They are run by licensed
    Facilitators in many countries around the world. To find
    a Facilitator, visit GoddessPlayshops.com

33 You can find the health magazine, Prevention, and take part in many quizzes online at prevention.com .

34 Edelman S, Rémond L (2005). Taking Charge! A Guide for Teenagers: Practical Ways to Overcome Stress, Hassles and Upsetting Emotions. Foundation for Life Sciences: fls.org.au

35 Reach Out! is a web-based service that inspires young people to help themselves through tough times. reachout.com.au

36 Share this 'Fall In Self-Love' piece with your friends from an excerpt published at SelfLoveAffair.com

37 Dove commissioned a study about unrealistic standards of beauty, and built a marketing campaign for healthy body image around it. campaignforrealbeauty.ph/flat3.asp?id=7089

38 Many of these tools are borrowed from The 7-Day Chakra Workout, which is available as a free e-Course from ChakraGoddess.com

39 The World Wide Essence Society (WWES) is a non-commercial organisation of vibrational/flower essence educators, practitioners, manufacturers, and distributors. Visit essences.com/wwes/

40 Natalie Maisel's work is housed at her website, GoddessDownload.com

41 Create your Goddess Creed: MyGoddessCreed.com

42 Janine Allis is the CEO of Boost Juice which she founded in response to growing demand for health takeaway food. boostjuicebars.com

43 David Cameron-Smith is an associate professor in nutrition sciences at Deakin University, Melbourne deakin.edu.au/hmnbs/ens/index.php